Praise for *THE PALEO DIET*

"*The Paleo Diet* helps you lose fat, improve your health, and feel great. Why? Because the Paleo Diet works with your genetics to help you realize your natural birthright of vibrant health and wellness. My book's success is due in large part to the revolutionary solutions provided by Professor Loren Cordain and his Paleo Diet message."

—Robb Wolf, author of the bestselling *The Paleo Solution*

"Loren Cordain's extensive research demonstrates how modern westernized diets drastically depart from the original diet humans consumed for millions of years. In *The Paleo Diet* and *The Paleo Diet Cookbook*, Dr. Cordain shows how diets high in grains, dairy, vegetable oils, salt, and refined sugars are at odds with our genetic legacy and then shares his uncomplicated strategy for losing weight and getting healthy."

—Arthur De Vany, Ph.D., author of *The New Evolution Diet*

"We found Dr. Loren Cordain's scientific research indispensable when we wrote *The 30-Day Low-Carb Diet Solution*. Cordain provides the most compelling arguments we've seen for why a protein-rich diet is the diet we were born to eat. His weight-loss plan simply works and his recipes are simply terrific."

—Michael R. Eades, M.D., and Mary Dan Eades, M.D., authors of *Protein Power, The 6-Week Cure for the Middle-Aged Middle*, and *The Low-Carb Comfort Food Cookbook*

"*The Paleo Diet* is at once revolutionary and intuitive. Its prescription provides without a doubt the most nutritious diet on the planet. Beautifully written, *The Paleo Diet* takes us from the theory to the day-to-day practice of the native human diet."

—Jennie Brand-Miller, Ph.D., coauthor of the bestselling The Glucose Revolution series

The Paleo Diet

REVISED EDITION

Lose Weight and Get Healthy by Eating
the Foods You Were Designed to Eat

Loren Cordain, Ph.D.

WILEY

John Wiley & Sons, Inc.

Published by John Wiley & Sons, Inc., Hoboken, New Jersey
Published simultaneously in Canada

The information contained in this book is not intended to serve as a replacement for professional medical advice. Any use of the information in this book is at the reader's discretion. The author and the publisher specifically disclaim any and all liability arising directly or indirectly from the use or application of any information contained in this book. A health care professional should be consulted regarding your specific situation.

For general information about our other products and services, please contact our Customer Care Department within the United States at (800) 762–2974, outside the United States at (317) 572–3993 or fax (317) 572–4002.

Wiley also publishes its books in a variety of electronic formats. Some content that appears in print may not be available in electronic books. For more information about Wiley products, visit our web site at www.wiley.com.

ISBN 978-0-470-91302-4 (paper); ISBN 978-1-118-00129-5 (ebk);
ISBN 978-1-118-00130-1 (ebk); ISBN 978-1-118-00131-8 (ebk)

Printed in the United States of America

10 9 8

To Lorrie, Kyle, Kevin, and Kenny
for making it all worthwhile

Contents

Preface to the Revised Edition

The original version of *The Paleo Diet* first came into print in January 2002. After its initial release, my book gained popularity and sales were good for the next few years, but it did not achieve chart-topping levels and the national exposure for which I had hoped. Fast-forward eight years to 2010: *The Paleo Diet* has become one of America's best-selling diet and health books.

This kind of sales history is almost unheard of in the publishing industry for successful diet books, which typically act like dwarf stars—they burn brightly at first and then fade away. Not so for *The Paleo Diet*, which started as a gentle glow and over the years has become hotter and hotter until now it is red hot. A diet book that once began as a ripple is now approaching tidal wave proportions.

Why? What is different about *The Paleo Diet* in 2010 compared to 2002? The material in the book has not radically changed, but the world has radically changed since 2002, particularly how we now communicate and inform one another about our lives, our daily experiences, and our reality. And herein is a clue to my book's sustained and increasing popularity.

When I first started to write *The Paleo Diet* in 2000, the Internet was in its youthful throes (Google had been founded only two years earlier, in 1998), and most people still used telephones (not cell phones) to talk. The U.S. Postal Service remained healthy because Bill Gates's foundational maxim "a personal computer in every household" had not yet taken firm hold, and snail mail reigned supreme. Then, "spam" simply meant canned meat. In the era of my book's baptism, texting, blogs, Facebook, YouTube, and most of the other Internet and electronic wizardry we now routinely take for granted still lay in the future. Then, people found out about the world through newspapers, radio, TV, and weekly news magazines. Now, except for the *New York Times* and a few other mainstays, daily newspapers have dried up to a trickle. Who wants to hear about outdated weekly news in paid-for magazines when you can get it for free and instantly from the Internet anytime you want? Like newspapers and magazines, radio and TV are not nearly as convenient or as timely as the Web—you can get Web versions of these media, anyway—so why bother with the real things?

When I wrote *The Paleo Diet* a decade ago, electronic interconnectedness was primitive, slow, and noninclusive. Local U.S. news was unavailable, obscure, or unknown in places like Uzbekistan or Botswana and vice versa. In those days, scientists reported new discoveries in their specialized journals, but this information was rarely picked up by newspapers or the popular press. It took years or decades for many discoveries to have an impact on people's lives. A decade ago, most people didn't argue with their physicians' diagnoses and prescriptions because "the doctor always knew best"—presumably because, then, the doctor was better informed than the patient was.

The Internet, Web sites, blogs, cell phones, and other various types of electronic wizardry have transformed our world within a mere decade or less. The electronic transmission of news and information and practical data to improve our lives, our financial situations, and our health has become humankind's universal language. Anyone in the world who has access to either a computer or a cell phone can immediately connect with anyone else who has the same technology. We now can and do talk to one another in unprecedented numbers—by the billions. A local event can instantaneously become a worldwide happening. Today what your next-door neighbor knows is available not only to you and your close friends, but literally to the world.

With such vast and nearly total information connectiveness, a subtle but crucial upshot of this brave new electronic world has arisen. When someone comes up with an answer to a complex or even a simple problem that is correct and that works, it gains followers like a snowball rolling downhill. Such has been the case for *The Paleo Diet*. It simply works. In an earlier era, prior to the Web, when human networks were small and noninclusive, information flowed slowly or not at all. Accordingly, correct answers sometimes smoldered for years, decades, or longer before they became widely recognized and accepted. Fortunately, *The Paleo Diet* came of age at the same time that the Internet was being adopted globally.

Had I originally written about a diet—a lifetime way of eating—that didn't work, *The Paleo Diet* would have simply faded into oblivion in the ensuing eight years since its publication. Yet it didn't. My book continues to gain more and more supporters as people like you relate their personal health experiences with *The Paleo Diet* to one another via the largest and most comprehensive human network ever created: the Internet. If *The Paleo Diet* had caused you to gain weight, made you feel lethargic, raised your blood cholesterol, promoted ill health, and been impossible to follow, it would have fallen by the wayside like most other dietary schemes dreamed up by human beings. Yet it didn't. In fact, *The Paleo Diet* movement continues to spread worldwide, thanks in part to the Web.

When people find correct answers to complex diet/health questions, they let their friends know, and thanks to the Internet, the momentum has accelerated. In the United States, the word "Paleo" has become part of mass culture, due in part to its popularity with the national CrossFit movement that is sweeping the country and recent coverage in the *New York Times*, the *Washington Post*, and other global media. *The Paleo Diet* has found wide acceptance not only with CrossFitters and athletes, but also with the medical and health professions, who have embraced it because of its wide-reaching therapeutic effects on metabolic syndrome diseases, autoimmune diseases, mental disorders, and beyond. In fact, there are very few chronic illnesses or diseases that do not respond favorably to our ancestral diet.

The novelty of *The Paleo Diet* is that a mortal human being like me didn't create it. Rather, I—along with many other scientists, physicians, and anthropologists worldwide—simply uncovered what was already there: the diet to which our species is genetically adapted. This is the diet of our hunter-gatherer ancestors, the foods consumed by every human being on the planet until a mere 333 human generations ago, or about ten thousand years ago. Our ancestors' diets were uncomplicated by agriculture, animal husbandry, technology, and processed foods. Then, as today, our health is optimized when we eat lean meats, seafood, and fresh fruits and veggies at the expense of grains, dairy, refined sugars, refined oils, and processed foods.

Nutritional science is not static. What we once believed to be true ten years ago is invariably replaced by fresh knowledge based on better experiments, more comprehensive data, and a newer understanding of how our bodies work. When I first wrote *The Paleo Diet*, a great deal of the dietary advice I offered was cutting edge— so much so, that it was looked on with skepticism by scientists and the public at large. Here's a perfect example. One 2002 online review of *The Paleo Diet* read, "Claims of improving diseases from diabetes to acne to polycystic ovary disease may be a little over-stated." I feel vindicated knowing that the original dietary recom-mendations I made for type 2 diabetes, acne, and polycystic ovary syndrome have been confirmed by hundreds of scientific experi-ments.

Especially gratifying are a series of epidemiological experiments from Dr. Walter Willett and colleagues at the Harvard School of Public Health that linked milk consumption and the occurrence of acne. Even more convincing evidence for the diet-acne link comes from Dr. Neil Mann's research group at the Royal Melbourne Insti-tute of Technology, where acne patients were actually fed high-protein, low-glycemic-load diets and reported significant improve-ment in their symptoms.

Anytime a diet/health book survives eight years, the hindsight rule (hindsight is 20/20) surely has to come into play. Indeed it did with this book, as reflected by my current updates and edits to the original volume. The elegance of *The Paleo Diet* concept is that the essential idea (the evolutionary basis for optimal human nutrition) is fundamentally sound and will never change; as Boyd Eaton, the godfather of Paleolithic nutrition commented, "The science behind Paleolithic Nutrition is indisputable; however, we will continually hone the concept as newer information accumulates."

So, what's new in this edition, and what are the noteworthy changes?

The first revision involves recommended oils. We are now down to only four: olive oil, flaxseed oil, walnut oil, and avocado oil. I no longer can recommend canola oil at all, and the only oil I believe should be used for cooking is olive oil. My friend and noted nutri-tionist Robert Crayhon always said to "let the data speak for itself," and I believe his words ring true. The rationale for these new rec-ommendations is solely based on new facts that have emerged. You can find this updated information in this revised edition.

Another shift is that I have softened my stance on the saturated fat issue as more and more data become available, including infor-mation from my recent evolutionary paper on the topic.

Finally, as scientists begin to unravel the mystery of autoimmune diseases, it is becoming apparent that multiple nutritional elements of the Paleo Diet may protect us from these one hundred or more illnesses that afflict nearly 10 percent of the U.S. population.

All of this information, along with the tweaks needed to bring *The Paleo Diet* up to date in 2010, is to be found within this edition. I've also just published a new book, *The Paleo Diet Cookbook*, which contains more than 150 Paleo recipes. I owe a debt of gratitude to each and every Paleo Diet supporter for making this concept known to the world.

Acknowledgments

I am the storyteller, but the tale I tell would not have been possible without the dedication and lifework of countless scientists from many diverse fields. I am particularly indebted to my friend and colleague S. Boyd Eaton for enlightening me with his seminal *New England Journal of Medicine* article "Paleolithic Nutrition" and then for generously recognizing me in the midst of a sea of faces. I have had countless hours of discussion (both on and off the electronic ether) regarding diet, disease, and anthropology with many notable scientists, physicians, and interested lay scholars. Without their encouragement, passion, knowledge, and enthusiasm, I suspect that this book would not have been written. Thank you, Boyd Eaton, Jennie Brand Miller, Neil Mann, Andy Sinclair, Mike and Mary Dan Eades, Artemis Simopoulous, Bruce Watkins, Dean Esmay, Ward Nicholson, Don Wiss, Ben Balzer, Clark Spencer Larsen, Mike Richards, John Speth, Norman Salem, Joe Hibbeln, Stephen Cunnane, Kim Hill, Craig Stanford, Robert Crayhon, Robert Gotshall, Joe Friel, Kevin Davy, Lynn Toohey, David Jenkins, David Lugwig, Soren Toubro, George Williams, Luisa Raijman, Michael Crawford, Staffan Lindeberg, Ray Audette, Wolfgang Lutz, Ann Magennis, Art DeVany, Ashton Embry, Bill DiVale, Pat Gray, Charlie Robbins, Irvin Liener, Nicolai Worm, Tony Sebastian, Robert Heaney, Stewart Truswell, and Pam Keagy. Finally, many thanks to my agents, Carol Mann and Channa Taub, for working indefatigably to get this book off the ground, and to my editor, Tom Miller, for his commitment to and enthusiasm for the Paleo Diet as a book concept.

PART ONE

Understanding the Paleo Diet

Introduction

This book represents the culmination of my lifelong interest in the link between diet and health, and of my fascination with anthropology and human origins. Although these scientific disciplines may at first appear to be unrelated, they are intimately connected. Our origins—the very beginnings of the human species—can be traced to pivotal changes in the diet of our early ancestors that made possible the evolution of our large, metabolically active brains. The Agricultural Revolution and the adoption of cereal grains as staple foods allowed us to abandon forever our previous hunter-gatherer lifestyle and caused the Earth's population to balloon and develop into the vast industrial-technological society in which we live today.

The problem, as you will see in this book, is that we are genetically adapted to eat what the hunter-gatherers ate. Many of our health problems today are the direct result of what we do—and do not—eat. This book will show you where we went wrong—how the standard American diet and even today's so-called healthy diets wreak havoc with our Paleolithic (Old Stone Age) constitutions. It will also show you how you can lose weight and regain health and well-being by eating the way our hunter-gatherer ancestors ate—the diet that nature intended.

The reason for this book is very simple: the Paleo Diet is the one and only diet that ideally fits our genetic makeup. Just 333 generations ago—and for 2.5 million years before that—every human being on Earth ate this way. It is the diet to which all of us are ideally suited and the lifetime nutritional plan that will normalize your weight and improve your health. I didn't design this diet—nature did. This diet has been built into our genes.

More than twenty years ago, I read a book that endorsed vegetarian dieting titled *Are You Confused?* I suspect that this title pretty much sums up how many of us feel about the conflicting breakthroughs and mixed messages we hear every day from scientific and medical authorities on what we should and shouldn't eat to lose weight and be healthy.

But here's the good news. Over the last twenty-five years, scientists and physicians worldwide have begun to agree on the fundamental principle underlying optimal nutrition—thanks in part to my colleague Dr. S. Boyd Eaton of Emory University in Atlanta. In 1985, Dr. Eaton published a revolutionary scientific paper called "Paleolithic Nutrition" in the prestigious *New England Journal of Medicine* suggesting that the ideal diet was to be found in the nutritional practices of our Stone Age ancestors. Although a few physicians, scientists, and anthropologists had been aware of this concept, it was Dr. Eaton's writings that brought this idea to center stage.

Dr. Eaton applied the most fundamental and pervasive idea of all biology and medicine—the theory of evolution by natural selection—to diet and health. His premise was simple: our genes determine our nutritional needs. And our genes were shaped by the selective pressures of our Paleolithic environment, including the foods our ancient ancestors ate.

Many modern foods are at odds with our genetic makeup—which, as we'll discuss in the book, is basically the same as that of our Paleolithic ancestors—and this is the cause of many of our modern diseases. By restoring the food types that we are genetically programmed to eat, we can not only lose weight, but also restore our health and well-being.

I have studied diet and health for the past three decades and have devoted the last twenty years to studying the Paleo Diet concept. I have been fortunate enough to work with Dr. Eaton to refine this groundbreaking idea and explore a wealth of new evidence. Together with many of the world's top nutritional scientists and anthropologists, I have been able to determine the dietary practices of our hunter-gatherer ancestors. Understanding what they ate is essential for understanding what we should eat today to improve our health and promote weight loss. Our research has been published in the top nutritional journals in the world.

It's all here for you in this book—all the dietary knowledge and wisdom that my research team and I have gleaned from our distant ancestors who lived in the days before agriculture. Part One explains what our Paleolithic ancestors ate, the basics of the Paleo Diet, and how civilization has made us stray from our original diet, bringing us ill health and obesity. Part Two shows how you can lose weight and how much you can lose, and also how the Paleo Diet can prevent and heal disease. Part Three spells out everything you need to know to follow the Paleo Diet—including meal plans for the three levels of the diet and more than 100 delicious Paleo recipes. That's the best part of the Paleo Diet—you'll eat well, feel great, and lose weight! The book ends with a complete list of scientific references that back up all of this information.

How Our Healthy Way of Life Went Wrong

The Agricultural Revolution began 10,000 years ago—just a drop in the bucket compared to the 2.5 million years that human beings have lived on Earth. Until that time—just 333 generations ago—everyone on the planet ate lean meats, fresh fruits, and vegetables. For most of us, it's been fewer than 200 generations since our ancestors abandoned the old lifestyle and turned to agriculture. If you happen to be an Eskimo or a Native American, it's been barely four to six generations. Except for perhaps a half-dozen tiny tribes in South America and a few on the Andaman Islands in the Bay of Bengal, pure hunter-gatherers have vanished from the face of the Earth. When these few remaining tribes become Westernized during the next decade or so, this ancient way of life—which allowed our species to thrive, grow, and mature—will come to an end.

This loss of humanity's original way of life matters a great deal. Why? Look at us. We're a mess. We eat too much, we eat the wrong foods, and we're fat. Incredibly, more Americans are overweight than aren't: 68 percent of all American men over age twenty-five, and 64 percent of women over age twenty-five are either overweight or obese. And it's killing us. The leading cause of death in the United States—responsible for 35 percent of all deaths or 1 of every 2.8 deaths—is heart and blood vessel disease. Seventy-three million Americans have high blood pressure; 34 million have high cholesterol levels, and 17 million have type 2 diabetes. It's not a pretty picture.

Most people don't realize just how healthy our Paleolithic ancestors were. They were lean, fit, and generally free from heart disease and the other ailments that plague Western countries. Yet many people assume that Stone Age people had it rough, that their lives were "poor, nasty, brutish, and short," as Thomas Hobbes wrote in *The Leviathan*.

But the historical and anthropological record simply does not support this line of reasoning. Almost without exception, descriptions of hunter-gatherers by early European explorers and adventurers showed these people to be healthy, fit, strong, and vivacious. These same characteristics can be yours when you follow the dietary and exercise principles I have laid out in the Paleo Diet.

I have examined thousands of early-nineteenth and twentieth-century photographs of hunter-gatherers. They invariably show indigenous people to be lean, muscular, and fit. The few medical studies of hunter-gatherers who managed to survive into the twentieth century also confirm earlier written accounts by explorers and frontiersmen. No matter where they lived—in the polar regions of Canada, the deserts of Australia, or the rain forests of Brazil—the medical records were identical. These people were free from signs and symptoms of the chronic diseases that currently plague us. And they were lean and physically fit. The medical evidence shows that their body fat, aerobic fitness, blood cholesterol, blood pressure, and insulin metabolism were always superior to those of the average modern couch potato. In most cases, these values were equivalent to those of modern-day, healthy, trained athletes.

High blood pressure (hypertension) is the most prevalent risk factor for heart disease in the United States. It's almost unheard of in indigenous populations. The Yanomamo Indians of northern Brazil and southern Venezuela, to whom salt was unknown in the late 1960s and early 1970s, were absolutely free from hypertension. Their blood pressure didn't increase with age and remained remarkably low by today's standards. Amazingly, scientific studies of Greenland Eskimos by Drs. Hans Bang and Jørn Dyerberg from Aalborg Hospital in Aalborg, Denmark, showed that despite a diet containing more than 60 percent animal food, not one death from heart disease—or even a single heart attack—occurred in 2,600 Eskimos from 1968 to 1978. This death rate from heart disease is one of the lowest ever reported in the medical literature. For a similar group of 2,600 people in the United States during a ten-year period, the expected number of deaths from heart disease would be about twenty-five.

When you put into practice the nutritional guidelines of the Paleo Diet, you will be getting the same protection from heart disease that the Eskimos had. You will also become lean and fit, like your ancient ancestors. This is your birthright. By going backward in time with your diet, you will actually be moving forward. You'll be combining the ancient dietary wisdom with all of the health advantages that modern medicine has to offer. You will reap the best of both worlds.

1

Not Just Another
Low-Carb Diet

What's the diet craze this week? You name it, there's a book selling it—and people buying it, hoping for a "magic bullet" to help them shed excess pounds. But how can everybody be right? More to the point, is *anybody* right? What are we supposed to eat? How can we lose weight, keep it off—and not feel hungry all the time? What's the best diet for our health and well-being?

For more than thirty years, as an avid researcher of health, nutrition, and fitness, I have been working to answer these questions. I started this quest because I wanted to get past all the hype, confusion, and political posturing swirling around dietary opinion. I was looking for facts: the simple, unadulterated truth. The answer, I found, was hidden back in time—way back, with ancient humans who survived by hunting wild animals and fish and gathering wild fruits and vegetables. These people were known as "hunter-gatherers," and my research team and I published our analysis of what many of them (more than 200 separate societies) ate in *The American Journal of Clinical Nutrition*. We were astonished at the diversity of their diet. We were also amazed at what they did *not* eat—which we'll get to in a minute and which may surprise you.

Health Secrets of Our Ancestors

What do Paleolithic people have to do with us? Actually, quite a lot: DNA evidence shows that basic human physiology has changed

9

little in 40,000 years. Literally, we are Stone Agers living in the Space Age; our dietary needs are the same as theirs. Our genes are well adapted to a world in which all the food eaten daily had to be hunted, fished, or gathered from the natural environment—a world that no longer exists. Nature determined what our bodies needed thousands of years before civilization developed, before people started farming and raising domesticated livestock.

In other words, built into our genes is a blueprint for optimal nutrition—a plan that spells out the foods that make us healthy, lean, and fit. Whether you believe the architect of that blueprint is God, or God acting through evolution by natural selection, or by evolution alone, the end result is still the same: We need to give our bodies the foods we were originally designed to eat.

Your car is designed to run on gasoline. When you put diesel fuel into its tank, the results are disastrous for the engine. The same principle is true for us: We are designed to run best on the wild plant and animal foods that all human beings gathered and hunted just 333 generations ago. The staples of today's diet—cereals, dairy products, refined sugars, fatty meats, and salted, processed foods—are like diesel fuel to our bodies' metabolic machinery. These foods clog our engines, make us fat, and cause disease and ill health.

Sadly, with all of our progress, we have strayed from the path designed for us by nature. For instance:

- Paleolithic people ate no dairy food. Imagine how difficult it would be to milk a wild animal, even if you could somehow manage to catch one.
- Paleolithic people hardly ever ate cereal grains. This sounds shocking to us today, but for most ancient people, grains were considered starvation food at best.
- Paleolithic people didn't salt their food.
- The only refined sugar Paleolithic people ate was honey, when they were lucky enough to find it.
- Wild, lean animal foods dominated Paleolithic diets, so their protein intake was quite high by modern standards, while their carbohydrate consumption was much lower.
- Virtually all of the carbohydrates Paleolithic people ate came from nonstarchy wild fruits and vegetables. Consequently, their carbohydrate intake was much lower and their fiber intake much higher than those obtained by eating the typical modern diet.

- The main fats in the Paleolithic diets were healthful, mono-unsaturated, polyunsaturated, and omega 3 fats—not the trans fats and certain saturated fats that dominate modern diets.

With this book, we are returning to the diet we were geneti-cally programmed to follow. The Paleo Diet is more than a blast from the past. It's the key to *speedy weight loss, effective weight control, and, above all, lifelong health.* The Paleo Diet enlists the body's own mechanisms, evolved over millions of years, to put the brakes on weight gain and the development of the chronic diseases of civili-zation. It is the closest approximation we can make, given the cur-rent scientific knowledge, to humanity's original, universal diet—the easy-to-follow, cravings-checking, satisfying program that nature itself has devised.

The Problems with Most Low-Carb Diets

The Paleo Diet is a low-carbohydrate diet—but that's where any resemblance to the glut of low-carbohydrate fad diets ends. Remember, the Paleo Diet is the only diet based on millions of years of nutritional facts—the one ideally suited to our biological needs and makeup and the one that most closely resembles hunter-gatherer diets. How does the Paleo Diet compare with the low-carb fad diets and the average U.S. diet?

Diet	Protein	Carbohydrate	Fat
The Paleo diet	19–35%	22–40%	28–47%
Typical U.S. diet	15.5%	49%	34%
Low-carb fad diets	18–23%	4–26%	51–78%

Modern low-carbohydrate weight-loss diets are really high-fat diets that contain moderate levels of protein. They don't have the high levels of protein that our ancestors ate—the levels found in the Paleo Diet. Actually, compared with what our ancestors ate, the carbohydrate content of these modern weight-loss diets is far too low. Even worse, almost all of these low-carbohydrate diets permit unlimited consumption of fatty, salty processed meats (such as bacon, sausage, hot dogs, and lunch meats) and dairy products (cheeses, cream, and butter) while restricting the consumption of fruits and vegetables. Cancer-fighting fruits and vegetables! This dietary pattern is drastically different from that of our ancestors.

And although low-carbohydrate diets may be successful in promoting weight loss, many dieters are achieving short-term weight loss at the expense of long-term health and well-being. Here's what the sellers of these diet plans don't want you to know: when low-carbohydrate diets cause weight loss in the short term, it's because they deplete the body's reserves of muscle and liver glycogen (carbohydrate), and the weight you're losing rapidly is mostly water weight.

When low-carbohydrate diets cause weight loss in the long run (weeks or months), it's because more calories are being burned than consumed, plain and simple. Low-carbohydrate diets tend to normalize insulin metabolism in many people, particularly in those who are seriously overweight. This normalization prevents swings in blood sugar that, in turn, may cause some people to eat less and lose weight. It is the cutback in total calories that lowers total cholesterol and low-density lipoprotein (LDL) cholesterol (the bad cholesterol) levels. Also, reductions in dietary carbohydrates (whether calories are cut or not) almost always cause a decline in blood triglycerides and an increase in blood high-density lipoprotein (HDL) cholesterol (the good cholesterol).

So, if low-carbohydrate diets cause someone to consume fewer calories, they may help produce weight loss and improvements in blood chemistry, at least over the short haul. However, dieters beware: when low-carbohydrate, high-fat diets are followed *without* a decrease in the daily consumption of calories, they are, according to the American Dietetic Association, "a nightmare." Let's see why.

Low Carb Doesn't Mean Low Cholesterol

Despite what anybody tells you—despite the outrageous claims of the low-carbohydrate, high-fat diet doctors—if you eat a lot of the saturated fats found in cheeses, butter, and bacon and don't cut your overall calorie intake, your cholesterol will go up. The medical community has known this for more than fifty years. It's been demonstrated in metabolic ward studies, in which people are locked into a hospital wing and only allowed to eat foods that have been carefully weighed and analyzed. Many of the low-carbohydrate diet doctors claim that these clinical trials are invalid because none of them reduced the carbohydrate content sufficiently. These doctors should know better; low carbohydrates don't guarantee low cholesterol.

Dr. Stephen Phinney and colleagues from the Massachusetts Institute of Technology conducted a normal caloric intake metabolic ward trial involving nine healthy, lean men. These men consumed nothing but meat, fish, eggs, cheese, and cream for thirty-five days. They had a low carbohydrate intake—less than 20 grams a day—but it didn't matter. Their blood cholesterol levels still went up, from 159 to 208 on average in just thirty-five days. This study indicates that diets high in a specific saturated fat called palmitic acid tends to raise blood cholesterol levels when caloric intake levels are normal.

So, at best, low-carbohydrate, high-fat diets are a temporary fix. At worst, they can cause big trouble in the long run by elevating LDL cholesterol levels, which increases the risk for heart and cardiovascular disease.

Healthy Fats, Not Lethal Fats

One major difference between the Paleo Diet and the low-carbohydrate, high-fat diets we just talked about is the fats. In most modern low-carbohydrate weight-loss diets, no distinction is made between good fats and bad fats. All fats are generally lumped together; the goal is simply to reduce carbohydrates and not worry about fats.

But you *should* worry about fats. Not all fats are created equal, and the impact of fat on blood cholesterol—and the odds of developing heart disease—can't be ignored. The problem is, fats are confusing for many people trying to make good dietary decisions. For one thing, many of them sound alike. How are saturated fats different from monounsaturated—or even polyunsaturated—fats? How are omega 6 fats different from the omega 3 variety?

- Monounsaturated fats are good. They're found in olive oil, nuts, and avocados; are known to lower blood cholesterol; and help prevent artery clogging or atherosclerosis.
- Saturated fats are mostly bad. They're found in processed meats, whole dairy products, and many bakery items; most of them are known to raise cholesterol. A key exception is a saturated fat called stearic acid, which, like monounsaturated fats, lowers blood cholesterol levels.
- Polyunsaturated fats are a mixed bag—some are more beneficial than others. For example, omega 3 polyunsaturated fats

(the kind found in fish oils) are healthy fats, which can improve blood chemistry and reduce your risk of many chronic diseases. But omega 6 polyunsaturated fats (found in vegetable oils, many baked goods, and snack foods) are not good when you eat too much of them at the expense of omega 3 fats.

People in the Paleolithic Age ate a lot of monounsaturated fats; they had saturated and polyunsaturated fats in moderation—but when they did have polyunsaturated fats, they had a proper balance of the omega 3 and omega 6 fats. They consumed far fewer omega 6 polyunsaturated fats than we do today. In addition, the main saturated fat in wild animals was healthful stearic acid, not the cholesterol-raising palmitic acid, which dominates the fat of feedlot cattle.

How important are fats in the diet? Here's a modern example: People who live in Mediterranean countries, who consume lots of olive oil, are much less likely to die of heart disease than Americans or northern Europeans, who don't consume as much olive oil. Instead, our Western diet is burdened by high levels of certain saturated fats, omega 6 fats, and trans fats and sadly lacking in heart-healthy, artery-protecting omega 3 fats.

Our studies of hunter-gatherers suggest that they had low blood cholesterol and relatively little heart disease. Our research team believes that dietary fats were a major reason for their freedom from heart disease.

Saturated Fats, Reconsidered

In the first edition of *The Paleo Diet*, I was adamant that you should avoid fatty processed meats such as bacon, hot dogs, lunch meats, salami, bologna, and sausages because they contain excessive saturated fats, which raise your blood cholesterol levels. That message still holds true today, but new information subtly alters this fundamental point of Paleo Dieting, and, as always, the devil lies in the details. Should you now go out and eat bacon and processed meats to your heart's desire? Absolutely not! Processed meats are synthetic mixtures of meat (muscle) and fat combined artificially at the meatpacker's or butcher's whim, with no regard for the true fatty acid profile of wild animal carcasses that our hunter-gatherer ancestors ate. In addition to their unnatural fatty acid profiles (high in omega 6 fatty acids, low in omega 3 fatty acids, and high in saturated fatty acids), processed fatty meats are full of preservatives such as nitrites, which are converted into potent cancer-causing nitrosamines in our guts. To make a bad situation worse, these unnatural meats are typically full of salt, high-fructose corn syrup, wheat, grains, and other additives that have multiple adverse health effects.

So, artificially produced, synthetic, factory meats have little or nothing to do with the wild animal foods our hunter-gatherer ancestors ate, and they should be avoided. But how about the unprocessed fatty meats that we routinely eat, day in and day out, that are produced in feedlots and butchered without adding fats or preservatives? These are meats such as T-bone steaks, spareribs, lamb chops, and chicken legs and thighs, as well as fatty cuts of pork and other fatty domestic meats. Are they a problem?

I realize that many, perhaps most, readers are not hunters and have never seen carcasses of wild animals, such as deer, elk, or antelope. Nor have you had the opportunity to visually contrast the carcasses of feedlot-produced animals to wild animals. I can tell you that there is no comparison. My research group and I have taken the time to do the chemical analyses between wild and feedlot-produced animals, and we have published our results in some of the top nutritional journals in the world.

Wild animal carcasses are lean, have little external fat, and exhibit virtually no fat between the muscles (marbling). In contrast, feedlot-produced cattle maintain a four- to six-inch layer of white fat covering the animal's entire body. These artificial products of modern agriculture are overweight, obese, and sick. Their muscles are infiltrated with that fat that we call marbling, a trait that improves flavor but makes the cattle insulin resistant and in poor health, just like us. Wild animals rarely or never exhibit marbling.

Because feedlot-raised animals are exclusively fed grains (corn and sorghum) in the last half of their lives, their meat has high concentrations of omega 6 fatty acids at the expense of health-promoting omega 3 fatty acids. The meat of grain-fed livestock is vastly at odds with that of wild animals. Check out Appendix B in this book. A 100 gram (~ ¼ lb.) serving of T-bone beefsteak gives you a walloping 9.1 grams of saturated fat, whereas a comparable piece of bison roast yields only 0.9 grams of saturated fat. You would have to eat ten times more bison meat to get a similar amount of saturated fat than the amount in a single serving of T-bone steak.

It would be difficult for our hunter-gatherer ancestors to eat anywhere near the amount of saturated fat that we get on a yearly basis in the typical Western diet. So, does dietary saturated fat promote heart disease? Should Paleo Dieters try to limit the fatty domesticated meats in their diet in order to reduce saturated fat? This question is not as clear-cut as it seemed twenty-five years ago, when Drs. Michael Brown and Joseph Goldstein of the University of Texas Southwest Medical Center were awarded the Nobel Prize in medicine for discovering that saturated fats down-regulated the LDL receptor. Their discovery and subsequent randomized, controlled human trials have unequivocally shown that certain saturated fats (lauric acid [12:0], myristic acid [14:0], and palmitic acid, [16:0]) but not all (stearic acid [18:0]), elevate blood cholesterol levels in humans, all other factors being equal. These facts are undeniable. Yet the next question is contentious and has divided the nutritional and medical community in recent years: do increased blood cholesterol levels necessarily predispose all people to an increased risk for cardiovascular disease?

As the scientific community has struggled with this question during the last few years, we should remember that the evolutionary template will almost always guide us to the correct answer. The clogging of arteries that eventually results in fatal heart attacks comes about through a process called atherosclerosis, in which plaque (cholesterol and calcium) builds up in the arteries that supply the heart itself with blood. It was originally thought that this buildup gradually narrowed and finally closed the arteries supplying the heart, thereby causing a heart attack. We now know that this model is inaccurate and too simple.

In the last ten to fifteen years, it has become apparent that inflammation is involved at every step of the way when arteries become clogged with plaque. In fact, the fatal event causing a heart attack is not the gradual narrowing of arteries supplying the heart but rather the rupturing of the fibrous cap that surrounds and walls off plaque that forms in the heart's arteries. Chronic low-level inflammation triggers the fibrous cap to rupture, which in turn causes a clot to form in the arteries that supply the heart, resulting in a heart attack. Without chronic low-level inflammation, heart attacks probably would rarely or never occur.

So, do dietary saturated fats from fatty meats cause the artery-clogging process known as atherosclerosis? If we look at the evolutionary evidence, the answer is a resounding yes. Dr. Michael

Zimmerman, a pathologist at Hahnemann University in Pennsylvania, had the rare opportunity to perform autopsies on a number of Eskimo mummies that had been frozen in Alaska's permafrost for hundreds of years. The first mummy was that of a fifty-three-year-old woman whose body washed out of the frozen banks of Saint Lawrence Island in October 1972. Radiocarbon dating indicated that she had died in 400 A.D. from a landslide that had completely buried her. Dr. Zimmerman's autopsy revealed moderate atherosclerosis in the arteries supplying her heart but no evidence of a heart attack. The second frozen mummy was also a female, forty to forty-five years of age, who had also been engulfed in an ice-and-mud-slide in 1520 A.D. near Barrow, Alaska. Similarly, the autopsy showed atherosclerotic plaques lining the arteries of her heart.

From my prior studies of worldwide hunter-gatherers, we know that these Eskimo women had a diet that consisted almost entirely (97 percent) of wild animal foods, including whales, walruses, seals, salmon, muskoxen, and caribou. Because they lived so far north (63 to 71 degrees north latitude), plant foods simply were unavailable; consequently, their carbohydrate intake was virtually zero. Yet they still developed atherosclerosis. Perhaps Drs. Brown and Goldstein were right, after all: high dietary intakes of saturated fats do promote atherosclerosis. Despite these facts, the best archaeological and medical evidence shows that Eskimos living and eating in their traditional ways rarely or never died from heart attacks or strokes.

So, now we have the facts we need to come to closure with the saturated fat–heart disease issue. Dietary saturated fats from excessive consumption of processed fatty meats and feedlot-produced meats increase our blood cholesterol concentrations, but unless our immune systems are chronically inflamed, atherosclerosis likely will not kill us from either heart attacks or strokes.

The new advice I can give you is this: If you are faithful to the basic principles of the Paleo Diet, consumption of fatty meats will probably have a minimal outcome on your health and well-being—as it did for our hunter-gatherer ancestors. Consumption of fatty meats and organs had survival value in an earlier time when humans didn't eat grains, legumes, dairy products, refined sugars, and salty processed foods, the foods that produce chronic low-level inflammation in our bodies through a variety of physiological mechanisms. I will explain this in more depth in my next book, *Living the Paleo Diet*.

Disease-Fighting Fruits and Vegetables

A big problem with low-carbohydrate weight-loss diets is what they do to health-promoting fruits and vegetables—they nearly eliminate them. Because of a technicality—a blanket restriction on all types of carbohydrates, even beneficial ones, to between 30 and 100 grams per day—fruits and veggies are largely off-limits. This is a mistake. Fruits and vegetables—with their antioxidants, phytochemicals, and fiber—are some of our most powerful allies in the war against heart disease, cancer, and osteoporosis. Yet just one papaya (59 grams of carbohydrate) would blow the daily limit for two of the most popular low-carbohydrate diets. Eating an orange, an apple, and a cup of broccoli and carrots (73 grams of carbohydrate)—just a drop in the bucket to hunter-gatherers, whose diets were rich in fruits and vegetables—would wreck all but the most liberal low-carbohydrate diets.

Humanity's original carbohydrate sources—the foods we survived on for millions of years—didn't come from starchy grains and potatoes, which have high glycemic indices that can rapidly cause blood sugar to spike. Instead, they came from wild fruits and vegetables with low glycemic indices that produced minimal, *gradual* rises in blood sugar. These are the carbohydrates that you'll be eating on the Paleo Diet. These nonstarchy carbohydrates normalize your blood glucose and insulin levels, promote weight loss, and make you feel energized all day long.

The Osteoporosis Connection

One of the greatest—and least recognized—benefits of fruits and vegetables is their ability to slow or prevent the loss of bone density, called "osteoporosis," that so often comes with aging. As far back as 1999, Dr. Katherine Tucker and colleagues at Tufts University examined the bone mineral status of a large group of elderly men and women. These scientists found that the people who ate the most fruits and vegetables had the greatest bone mineral densities and the strongest bones. In the ensuing ten years, more than 100 scientific studies have confirmed this concept.

But what about calcium? Surely, eating a lot of cheese can help prevent osteoporosis? The answer is a bit more complicated. One of the great ironies of the low-carbohydrate, high-fat diets is that even though they allow unlimited consumption of high-calcium cheeses, they almost certainly will be found to promote bone loss and osteoporosis in the long run. How can this be? Because getting a lot of dietary calcium from cheese, by itself, isn't enough to offset the lack of fruits and vegetables.

Nutrition scientists use the term "calcium balance" to describe this process. It's the difference between how much calcium you take in and how much you excrete. Most of us have gotten the message about consuming calcium. But the other part of the equation—*how much calcium you excrete*—is just as important. It is quite possible for you to be in calcium balance on a low calcium intake if your calcium excretion is also low. On the other hand, it's easy for you to fall out of calcium balance—even if you load up on cheese at every meal—if you lose more calcium than you take in.

The main factor that determines calcium loss is yet another kind of balance—the *acid-base balance*. If your diet has high levels of acid, you'll lose more calcium in your urine; if you eat more alkaline foods, you'll retain more calcium. A study in the *New England Journal of Medicine* by my colleague Dr. Anthony Sebastian and his research group at the University of California at San Francisco showed that simply taking potassium bicarbonate (an alkaline base) neutralized the body's internal acid production, reduced urinary calcium losses, and increased the rate of bone formation. In a follow-up report in the *New England Journal of Medicine*, Dr. Lawrence Appel at Johns Hopkins University reported that diets rich in fruits and vegetables (these are alkaline foods) significantly reduced urinary calcium loss in 459 men and women.

See Appendix A for a list of common foods and their acid-base values.

Cereals, most dairy products, legumes, meat, fish, salty processed foods, and eggs produce net acid loads in the body. By far the worst offenders on this list are the hard cheeses, which are rich sources of calcium. Again, unless you get enough fruits and vegetables, eating these acid-rich foods will actually promote bone loss and osteoporosis.

Virtually all fruits and vegetables produce alkaline loads in the body. When you adopt the Paleo Diet, you won't have to worry about excessive dietary acid causing bone loss—because you'll be getting 35 percent or more of your daily calories as healthful alkaline fruits and vegetables that will neutralize the dietary acid you get when you eat meat and seafood.

Toxic Salt

Most low-carbohydrate, high-fat diets don't address the dangers of salt; some even encourage its use. And yet there is a ton of medical evidence linking salt to high blood pressure, stroke, osteoporosis, kidney stones, asthma, and even certain forms of cancer. Salt is also implicated as a factor in insomnia, air and motion sickness, Ménière's syndrome (an agonizing ear ringing), and the preeclampsia of pregnancy.

Salt is made up of sodium and chloride. Although most people think that the sodium portion of salt is entirely responsible for most of its unhealthful effects, chloride is just as guilty, if not more so. The average American eats about 10 grams of salt a day (this turns out to be about 4 grams of sodium and 6 grams of chloride). Chloride, like cereals, dairy products, legumes, and meats, yields a net acid load to the kidneys after it is digested. Because of its high chloride content, salt is one of the worst offenders in making your diet more acid.

Paleolithic people hardly ever used salt and never ate anything like today's salty cheeses, processed meats, and canned fish advocated by most of the low-carbohydrate weight-loss diets. Do your body a favor and throw out your saltshaker along with all the highly salted, processed, packaged, and canned foods in your pantry.

Lean Meat Helps You Lose Weight

It's taken half a century, but scientists have finally realized that when they stigmatized red meat, they threw out the proverbial baby with the bathwater. Meat is a mixture of fat and protein. Lean meat—such as that found in wild game and seafood—is about 80 percent protein and about 20 percent fat. But fatty processed meats like bacon and hot dogs can pack a whopping 75 percent of their calories as fat and only 25 percent or less as protein. What should have been obvious—that it was the high level of a certain saturated fat, palmitic acid, not the protein, that caused health problems—was essentially ignored. Meat protein had unfairly become a villain.

Here again, there's a major lesson to be learned from looking at the distant past: for more than 2 million years, our ancestors had a diet rich in lean protein and healthful fats. It gave them energy and, combined with fruits and vegetables, helped them stay healthy.

Protein Increases Your Metabolism and Slows Your Appetite

When scientists actually studied how lean protein influences health, well-being, and body-weight regulation—and this has occurred only in the last two decades—they found that our ancestors were right all along. It turns out that *lean protein is perhaps our most powerful ally in the battle of the bulge.* It has twice the "thermic effect" of either fats or carbohydrates, which means it revs up your metabolism. In other words, protein's thermic effect increases our metabolism and causes us to burn more calories than if we ate an equal caloric serving of either fat or carbohydrate. Also, more than fats, more than carbohydrates, protein has the highest "satiating value"—that is, it does the best job of making us feel full.

The principles I have laid out in the Paleo Diet—all based on decades of scientific research and proved over millions of years by our ancestors—will make your metabolism soar, your appetite shrink, and extra pounds begin to melt away as you include more and more lean protein in your meals.

Lean Protein and Heart Disease

But this diet gives you much more than a slimmer figure. Unlike other low-carbohydrate diets, it's good for your heart. High-protein diets have been shown by Dr. Bernard Wolfe at the University of Western Ontario in Canada to be more effective than low-fat, high-carbohydrate diets in lowering total and bad LDL cholesterol and triglycerides while simultaneously increasing the good HDL cholesterol. My colleague Neil Mann at the Royal Melbourne Institute of Technology in Melbourne, Australia, has demonstrated that people who eat a lot of lean meat have lower blood levels of homocysteine (a toxic substance in the blood that damages the arteries and predisposes them to atherosclerosis) than do vegan vegetarians. The net result is that high-protein diets produce beneficial changes in your blood chemistry that, in turn, reduce your overall risk of heart disease.

High-protein diets have been shown to improve insulin metabolism, help lower blood pressure, and reduce the risk of stroke. They have even prolonged survival in women with breast cancer.

Some people have been told that high-protein diets damage the kidneys. They don't. Scientists at the Royal Veterinary and Agricultural University in Copenhagen effectively put this myth to rest. Dr. Arne Astrup and colleagues put sixty-five overweight people on a high-protein diet for six months and found that their kidneys easily adapted to increased protein levels. Furthermore, kidney function remained perfect at the end of the experiment.

Isn't it time you got protein on your side? Eating lean meat and fish at every meal, just as your Paleolithic ancestors did, could be the healthiest decision you ever made.

Compared to the faddish low-carbohydrate weight-loss diets, the Paleo Diet includes all the nutritional elements needed to encourage weight loss while promoting health and well-being. The Paleo Diet is designed to imitate the healthful diets of our pre-agricultural ancestors. It contains the proper balance of plant and animal foods—and the correct ratios of protein, fat, and carbohydrate required for weight loss and excellent health.

So, don't be fooled by the low-carbohydrate fad diets. The Paleo Diet gives you the same weight-loss benefits, but it's also a delicious, healthy diet you can maintain for a lifetime.

2

The Ground Rules
for the Paleo Diet

With the Paleo Diet, you'll be restoring the diet you are geneti-cally programmed to eat. You'll be following the diet that every single person on the planet ate only 333 generations ago. It is the diet the modern world has completely forgotten.

The Paleo Diet is simplicity itself. Here are the ground rules:

1. All the lean meats, fish, and seafood you can eat
2. All the fruits and nonstarchy vegetables you can eat
3. No cereals
4. No legumes
5. No dairy products
6. No processed foods

The Paleo Diet is not a fat-free diet, it's a "bad fat"–free diet. It has few of the artery-clogging fats found in the typical Western diet, but there is plenty of low-fat protein and good fats—such as those found in salmon and other cold-water fish, as well as in nuts and olive oil. It is not a fanatically strict diet, either.

There are three levels of adherence that make it easy to follow the diet's principles. Each level contains a limited number of Open Meals—in which you can still eat your favorite foods. If you enjoy an occasional glass of wine or beer, that's fine—it's allowed here. Because the Paleo Diet is a lifetime program of eating—and not a quick-fix weight-loss diet—it has built-in flexibility to accommo-date a little cheating and your own individuality.

Try it, and from the beginning your appetite will be reduced and your metabolism will be increased. This means you'll lose weight without the hunger pangs that accompany so many diets— and ultimately doom these diets to fail. There's no need to count carbohydrate grams in this diet. You can eat as much carbohydrate as you want, as long as it's the good kind—the kind that comes from low-glycemic fruits and vegetables. There is no need to count calories. This is how our diet was meant to be: Eat until you're full. Enjoy nature's bounty. Lose weight, and be healthy while you're doing it.

Here's how the Paleo Diet compares to the faddish low-carbohydrate diets we discussed in the previous chapter.

Item	The Paleo Diet	Fad Low-Carb Diets
Protein	High (19–35%)	Moderate (18–23%)
Carbohydrate	Moderate (22–40%)	Low (4–26%)
Total fat	Moderate (28–47%)	High (51–78%)
Saturated fat	Moderate	High
Monounsaturated fat	High	Moderate
Polyunsaturated fat	Moderate	Moderate
Omega 3 fat	High	Low
Total fiber	High	Low
Fruits and vegetables	High	Low
Nuts and seeds	Moderate	Low
Salt	Low	High
Refined sugars	Low	Low
Dairy foods	None	High

The Fundamentals of the Paleo Diet

The Paleo Diet is based on the bedrock of Stone Age diets:

Eat lots of lean meats, fresh fruits, and vegetables

From the work my research team and I have done in analyzing the daily food intake of hunter-gatherer societies, we have found the ideal dietary ratio. Although you don't need to count calories with the Paleo Diet, if you did you'd find that a little more than half— 55 percent—of your calories comes from lean meats, organ meats, fish, and seafood. The balance comes from fresh fruits and vegetables, some nuts, and healthful oils.

My research team and I have spent years analyzing what Paleolithic humans ate—running hundreds of computerized analyses exploring every conceivable dietary component, varying the amounts and types of plant and animal foods that were available to our ancient ancestors. No matter how we mixed up the ingredients, seven dietary characteristics consistently emerged. They are the Seven Keys of the Paleo Diet—your guidelines to weight loss and good health.

The Seven Keys of the Paleo Diet

1. Eat a relatively high amount of animal protein compared to that in the typical American diet.
2. Eat fewer carbohydrates than most modern diets recommend, but eat lots of good carbohydrates—from fruits and vegetables, not from grains, starchy tubers, and refined sugars.
3. Eat a large amount of fiber from nonstarchy fruits and vegetables.
4. Eat a moderate amount of fat, with more good (monounsaturated and polyunsaturated) fats than bad (trans and certain saturated) fats, and nearly equal amounts of omega 3 and omega 6 fats.
5. Eat foods with a high potassium content and a low sodium content.
6. Eat a diet with a net alkaline load.
7. Eat foods rich in plant phytochemicals, vitamins, minerals, and antioxidants.

The Seven Keys optimize health, minimize the risk of chronic disease, and cause excess weight to melt away. This is the way we're genetically programmed to eat.

Just the Foods You Can Hunt and Gather at Your Supermarket

You don't have to eat wild game meat (unless you want to) to achieve the same health benefits that kept the world's hunter-

gatherers free from the chronic diseases of civilization. The mainstays of the Paleo Diet are the lean meats, organ meats, and fish
and seafood that are available at your local supermarket.

Here are some high-protein foods that are part of the Paleo Diet:

- Skinless turkey breast (94 percent protein)
- Shrimp (90 percent protein)
- Red snapper (87 percent protein)
- Crab (86 percent protein)
- Halibut (80 percent protein)
- Beef sweetbreads (77 percent protein)
- Steamed clams (73 percent protein)
- Lean pork tenderloin (72 percent protein)
- Beef heart (69 percent protein)
- Broiled tuna (68 percent protein)
- Veal steak (68 percent protein)
- Sirloin beef steak (65 percent protein)
- Chicken livers (65 percent protein)
- Skinless chicken breasts (63 percent protein)
- Beef liver (63 percent protein)
- Lean beef flank steak (62 percent protein)
- Lean pork chops (62 percent protein)
- Mussels (58 percent protein)

Although you may think of hamburger, eggs, cheese, milk, and
legumes as high-protein foods, think again. None of these foods
can hold a candle to lean meat and fish when it comes to protein
content.

- Eggs (34 percent protein)
- Cheeses (28 percent protein)
- Legumes (27 percent protein)
- Lamb chops (25 percent protein)
- Fatty hamburger (24 percent protein)
- Dry salami (23 percent protein)
- Link pork sausage (22 percent protein)
- Bacon (21 percent protein)
- Whole milk (21 percent protein)
- Liverwurst sausage (18 percent protein)
- Bologna (15 percent protein)
- Hot dogs (14 percent protein)
- Cereal grains (12 percent protein)
- Nuts (10 percent protein)

You don't have to eat bone marrow (a favorite food of hunter-gatherers) on the Paleo Diet, either, but here's why it was good for our Paleolithic ancestors: marrow is a major source of monounsaturated fat—another good fat. Monounsaturated fats lower your cholesterol level and reduce your risk of breast cancer and heart disease. You can find monounsaturated fats in nuts, avocados, and olive oil.

Nor do you have to eat brains (another delicacy for hunter-gatherers) to get omega 3 fats—one of the good fats we talked about in chapter 1 and quite important in preventing many chronic diseases. You can get plenty of health-sustaining omega 3 fats from many foods found in the supermarket, such as:

- Fish and seafood, particularly cold-water fish such as salmon, mackerel, herring, and halibut
- Flaxseed oil, which can be used in several ways—as an ingredient in salad dressings, poured over steamed vegetables, or taken as a supplement
- Liver
- Game meat
- Free-range chickens
- Pasture-fed beef
- Eggs enriched with omega 3
- Salt-free walnuts and macadamia nuts (which are also tasty in salads)
- Leafy green vegetables
- Fish oil capsules, available at health food stores

Meal Preparation and Typical Meals

Eating unadulterated, healthful lean meats, seafood, fruits, and veggies at every meal requires a little bit of planning and foresight, but once you get into the swing of things, it will become second nature. Even working people who must eat away from home can easily incorporate real foods into their busy schedules; so can people who travel often or who must frequently dine out.

One of the keys to becoming a successful Paleo Dieter is to prepare some of your food at home and bring it with you to work either as a snack or as a meal. For lunch, nothing could be simpler than to brown-bag a few slices of last night's lean roast beef or skinless chicken breasts along with some fresh tomato wedges, a few carrot sticks, and an apple or a fresh peach.

Eating Paleo style while dining out is also quite easy if you follow a few simple guidelines. Order a tossed green salad with shrimp, but hold the croutons and dress it with olive oil and lemon juice. For breakfast out, try two poached eggs and half a cantaloupe, skip the toast and bacon, and treat yourself to a cup of decaffeinated coffee or herbal tea. In chapter 8, I fully outline how to pull off a Paleo Diet in our fast-food world.

Although you will be eliminating grains, dairy products, refined sugars, and processed foods from your daily fare, you will soon discover the incredible bounty and diversity of delicious and healthful foods that the Paleo Diet has to offer. How about a breakfast omelet made with omega 3–enriched eggs and stuffed with crab and avocado and covered with peach salsa? A filet of sole simmered in wine sauce accompanied by spinach salad and gazpacho soup for lunch? For dinner, does roast pork loin, a tossed green salad dressed with flaxseed oil, steamed broccoli, a glass of Merlot, and a bowl of fresh blackberries sprinkled with almond slices sound tempting? These are just a few of the six weeks' worth of meal plans and more than 100 Paleo recipes I provide you with in chapters 9 and 10.

The Paleo Diet: A Nutritional Bonanza

Many registered dietitians and knowledgeable nutritionists would predict that any diet that excludes all cereal grains, dairy products, and legumes would lack many important nutrients and would require extremely careful planning to make it work. Just the opposite is true with the Paleo Diet—which confirms yet again that this is exactly the type of diet human beings were meant to thrive on, as they have for all but the last 10,000 years.

The Paleo Diet provides 100 percent of our nutrient requirements. My research team has analyzed the nutrient composition of hundreds of varying combinations of the Paleo Diet, in which we've altered the percentage as well as the types of plant and animal foods it contains. In virtually every dietary permutation, the levels of vitamins and minerals exceed governmental recommended daily allowances (RDAs). The Paleo Diet even surpasses modern cereal- and dairy-based diets in many nutritional elements that protect against heart disease and cancer, including:

- Vitamin C
- Vitamin B$_{12}$

- Vitamin B_6
- Folic acid
- Magnesium
- Chromium
- Potassium
- Selenium
- Soluble fiber
- Omega 3 and monounsaturated fats
- Beta-carotene and other plant phytochemicals

In fact, the Paleo Diet is packed with much higher levels of many nutrients that are deficient in both vegetarian and average American diets, such as iron, zinc, vitamin B_{12}, vitamin B_6, and omega 3 fats.

Let's take a quick look at the daily nutrient intake of a twenty-five-year-old woman on the Paleo Diet. Out of a typical 2,200 calories, half come from animal foods and half from plant foods—all available at the supermarket.

For breakfast, she eats half a cantaloupe and a 12-ounce portion of broiled Atlantic salmon. Lunch is a shrimp, spinach/vegetable salad (seven large boiled shrimp, three cups of raw spinach leaves, one shredded carrot, one sliced cucumber, two diced tomatoes, lemon juice/olive oil/spice dressing). For dinner, she has two lean pork chops, two cups of steamed broccoli, and a tossed green salad (two cups of romaine lettuce, a half-cup of diced tomatoes, a quarter-cup of sliced purple onions, half an avocado, lemon juice dressing). She tops it all off with a half-cup of fresh or frozen blueberries and a quarter-cup of slivered almonds. For a snack, she has a quarter-cup of slivered almonds and a cold pork chop.

Nutrient	Daily Intake	RDA
Calories	2,200.0	100%
Protein	190.0 (g)	379%
Carbohydrate	142.0 (g)	—
Fat	108.0 (g)	—
Saturated fat	21.0 (g)	—
Monounsaturated fat	54.0 (g)	—
Polyunsaturated fat	21.0 (g)	—
Omega 3 fats	6.7 (g)	—
Water-soluble vitamins		
Thiamin (B_1)	4.6 (mg)	417%

Nutrient	Daily Intake	RDA
Riboflavin (B_2)	3.6 (mg)	281%
Niacin (B_3)	56.2 (mg)	374%
Pyridoxine (B_6)	5.9 (mg)	369%
Cobalamin (B_{12})	10.3 (μg)	513%
Biotin	113.0 (μg)	174%
Folate	911.0 (μg)	506%
Pantothenic acid	11.5 (mg)	209%
Vitamin C	559.0 (mg)	932%
Fat-soluble vitamins		
Vitamin A	6,861.0 (RE)	858%
Vitamin D	0.0 (μg)	0%
Vitamin E	26.5 (mg)	331%
Vitamin K	945.0 (μg)	1,454%
Macro minerals		
Sodium	813.0 (mg)	—
Potassium	8,555.0 (mg)	—
Calcium	890.0 (mg)	111%
Phosphorus	2,308.0 (mg)	289%
Magnesium	685.0 (mg)	245%
Trace minerals		
Iron	21.5 (mg)	143%
Zinc	19.8 (mg)	165%
Copper	3.5 (mg)	155%
Manganese	6.4 (mg)	181%
Selenium	0.147 (mg)	267%
Dietary fiber	47.0 (g)	—
Beta-carotene	3,583.0 (μg)	—

As you can see, the Paleo Diet is extremely nutritious. The macronutrient breakdown for this sample 2,200-calorie diet is 33 percent protein, 25 percent carbohydrate, and 42 percent fat. Note that for every nutrient except vitamin D, the daily nutrient intake ranges from 1.5 to more than 10 times the governmentally suggested RDA. Even "healthful" vegetarian diets don't reach these nutrient levels. The Paleo Diet is rich in antioxidant vitamins (A, C, and E), minerals (selenium), and plant phytochemicals, such as beta-carotene, which can help prevent the development of heart disease and cancer. In addition, the high levels of B vitamins (B_6, B_{12}, and folate) prevent elevated levels of blood homocysteine, a potent risk factor for atherosclerosis, and also have been associated with a reduced risk of colon cancer and spina bifida, a neural tube birth defect.

Even though the fat content (42 percent of total calories) is slightly higher than that in the average American diet (31 percent of total calories), these are good fats—healthful, cholesterol-lowering monounsaturated and polyunsaturated fats. Actually, the monounsaturated fat intake is twice that of saturated fat. As I discussed earlier, the high levels of omega 3 fats also help protect against heart disease by their ability to thin the blood, prevent fatal heartbeat irregularities, and lower blood triglycerides.

Not only does the Paleo Diet provide you with an abundance of nutrients, it's also extremely high in fiber. This, too, can lower blood cholesterol. It promotes normal bowel function and prevents constipation as well.

Finally, because extra salt and processed salty foods are not part of the Paleo Diet, the sodium (and chloride) content here is very low, while the potassium content is quite high. As we've discussed, this high-potassium/low-sodium balance helps prevent high blood pressure, kidney stones, asthma, osteoporosis, certain types of cancer, and other chronic diseases known to be associated with high-salt diets.

The amount of vitamin D you'll get on the Paleo Diet is negligible, because vitamin D is found only in trace quantities in all naturally occurring foods, except for fish liver oils. But we don't *need* to eat that much vitamin D—we can get all we need from the sun. (When we're exposed to ultraviolet radiation from sunlight, our bodies synthesize vitamin D from the cholesterol in our skin.) Our Paleolithic ancestors spent much of their time outdoors, and they manufactured all the vitamin D they needed from the sun's natural rays. Today, many of us get insufficient sunlight exposure to synthesize optimal levels of vitamin D. This is why milk, margarine, and other processed foods are fortified with vitamin D. We would all do well to incorporate some of the Stone Age lifestyle and make sure to get some daily sunshine. However, if your busy lifestyle doesn't allow it, particularly during short winter days, I recommend that you take a vitamin D supplement (at least 2,000 I.U./day).

Perhaps the most important element of the Paleo Diet is its high protein intake—nearly four times higher than the RDA. As I've discussed, this high level of protein helps you lose weight by increasing your metabolism and reducing your appetite. A 1999 clinical report in the *International Journal of Obesity* by my friend Dr. Soren Toubro and colleagues from the Royal Veterinary and Agricultural University in Copenhagen, Denmark, has shown that when it comes to weight loss, high-protein, low-calorie diets are much more effective than low-calorie, high-carbohydrate diets. In the ensuing eleven years, hundreds of scientific papers have confirmed these seminal results. Also, high levels of low-fat protein lower your cholesterol, reduce triglycerides and increase good HDL cholesterol, and reduce your risk of high blood pressure, stroke, and certain forms of cancer. When accompanied by sufficient amounts of alkaline fruit and vegetables, high-protein diets do not promote osteoporosis. Instead, they protect you from it.

The Typical American Diet: A Nutritional Nightmare

Now let's take a look at this same 2,200 calorie diet for our sample twenty-five-year-old woman—but let's replace most of the real foods (lean meats and fruits and vegetables) with processed foods, cereal grains, and dairy products. Remember, the U.S. Department of Agriculture (USDA) Food Pyramid encourages you to eat six to eleven servings of grains every day. The nutrient breakdown depicted below closely resembles that of the average American diet. This is the same diet that has produced a nation in which 68 percent of all American men over age twenty-five and 64 percent of women over age twenty-five are either overweight or obese.

For breakfast, our twenty-five-year-old woman eats a Danish pastry and two cups of cornflakes with 8 ounces of whole milk, topped off with a teaspoon of sugar, and drinks a cup of coffee with a tablespoon of cream and a teaspoon of sugar. Because of the large amounts of refined carbohydrates consumed for breakfast, her blood sugar level soon plummets and she is hungry again by midmorning, so she eats a glazed doughnut and drinks another cup of coffee with cream and sugar. By noon, she's hungry again. She goes to the McDonald's near her office and orders a Quarter Pounder, a small portion of French fries, and a 12-ounce cola drink. For dinner, she eats two slices of cheese pizza and a small iceberg lettuce salad with half a tomato, covered with two tablespoons of Thousand Island dressing. She washes it all down with 12 ounces of lemon-lime soda. Let's examine the nutrient breakdown of this dietary disaster:

Nutrient	Daily Intake	RDA
Calories	2,200.0	100%
Protein	62.0 (g)	57%
Carbohydrate	309.0 (g)	—
Fat	83.0 (g)	—
Saturated fat	29.0 (g)	—
Monounsaturated fat	19.0 (g)	—
Polyunsaturated fat	10.0 (g)	—
Omega 3 fats	1.0 (g)	—
Water-soluble vitamins		
Thiamin (B_1)	1.0 (mg)	95%
Riboflavin (B_2)	1.1 (mg)	87%
Niacin (B_3)	11.0 (mg)	73%
Pyridoxine (B_6)	0.3 (mg)	20%
Cobalamin (B_{12})	1.8 (µg)	88%
Biotin	11.8 (µg)	18%
Folate	148.0 (µg)	82%
Pantothenic acid	1.8 (mg)	32%
Vitamin C	30.0 (mg)	51%
Fat-soluble vitamins		
Vitamin A	425.0 (RE)	53%
Vitamin D	3.1 (µg)	63%
Vitamin E	2.7 (mg)	34%
Vitamin K	52.0 (µg)	80%
Macro minerals		
Sodium	2,943.0 (mg)	—
Potassium	2,121.0 (mg)	—
Calcium	887.0 (mg)	111%
Phosphorus	918.0 (mg)	115%
Magnesium	128.0 (mg)	46%
Trace minerals		
Iron	10.2 (mg)	68%
Zinc	3.9 (mg)	33%
Copper	0.4 (mg)	19%
Manganese	0.9 (mg)	28%
Selenium	0.040 (mg)	73%
Dietary fiber	8.0 (g)	—
Beta-carotene	87.0 (µg)	—

This diet typifies everything that's wrong with the way most of us eat today—the modern, processed food–based diet. It violates all of the Seven Keys of the Paleo Diet—the ones we're genetically programmed to follow. Except for calcium and phosphorus, every nutrient falls below the RDA. The protein intake on the standard American diet is a paltry 62 grams (57 percent of the RDA) compared to that of the Paleo Diet (a mighty 190 grams, or 379 percent of the RDA). Remember, protein is your ally in weight loss and good health. It lowers your cholesterol, improves your insulin sensitivity, speeds up your metabolism, satisfies your appetite, and helps you lose weight.

Even though there is very little meat in the typical American diet of this woman, the saturated fat content (29 grams) is 38 percent higher than that of the Paleo Diet. Worse still is the mix of fats. Healthful, cholesterol-lowering polyunsaturated and mono-unsaturated fats total a meager 29 grams. (In contrast, they add up to 75 grams on the Paleo Diet.) There is only 1 gram of heart-healthy omega 3 fats for the whole day in the typical American diet compared to a bountiful 6.7 grams in the sample Paleo Diet meal. Is it any wonder that the cereal-based, processed food–laden American diet promotes heart disease?

Now take a look at vitamin B_6 (20 percent of the RDA), vitamin B_{12} (88 percent of the RDA), and folate (82 percent of the RDA). This woman's diet is deficient in all three of the vitamins that prevent toxic buildup of homocysteine, the substance that damages the arteries and further predisposes you to heart disease. Inadequate amounts of folate also increase the risk of colon cancer and the birth defect spina bifida.

It's also worth noting that this sample American diet has three times more sodium—but four times less potassium—than the Paleo Diet. This mineral imbalance promotes or aggravates conditions and diseases due to acid-base imbalance, including high blood pressure, osteoporosis, kidney stones, asthma, stroke, and certain forms of cancer. The daily intake of magnesium is also quite low here (46 percent of the RDA). Numerous scientific studies have shown that having a low magnesium level puts you at risk for heart disease by elevating your blood pressure, increasing your cholesterol level, and predisposing your heart to irregular beats. A low intake of magnesium also promotes the formation of kidney stones.

A high intake of antioxidant vitamins and phytochemicals

from fresh fruits and vegetables is one of the best dietary strategies you can adopt to reduce the risk of cancer and heart disease. Unfortunately, when cereals, dairy products, processed foods, and fatty meats displace fruits and vegetables, they automatically lower your intake of health-giving antioxidants and phytochemicals from fruits and veggies. There is no comparison between the RDA percentages of vitamin A (53 percent), vitamin C (51 percent), vitamin E (34 percent), and selenium (73 percent) in the example above and those in the Paleo Diet: vitamin A (858 percent), vitamin C (932 percent), vitamin E (331 percent), and selenium (267 percent). The Paleo Diet contains forty-one times more beta-carotene (a natural plant antioxidant) than the average American diet.

The average American diet is also deficient in zinc (33 percent of the RDA) and iron (68 percent of the RDA)—which, along with a low intake of vitamins A and C, can impair your immune system and open the door to colds and infections.

Because the average American diet is loaded with refined cereal grains (six servings in our example) and sugars (123 grams or about a quarter-pound in our example), it increases the blood sugar and insulin levels in many people. If insulin remains constantly elevated, it causes a condition known as hyperinsulinemia, which increases the risk of a collection of diseases called metabolic syndrome—type 2 diabetes, high blood pressure, high cholesterol, obesity, and harmful changes in blood chemistry. But refined cereals and sugars are not part of the Paleo Diet—which means that your dietary insulin level will be naturally low and you will automatically reduce your risk of metabolic syndrome diseases. Last but not least is fiber. The average American diet contains a measly 8 grams compared to 47 grams on the Paleo Diet.

Many nutritionists would say that the example diet is healthful because it contains large amounts of carbohydrate (55 percent of total calories) and a low total fat intake (34 percent of total calories). This is also the message that most Americans have heard loud and clear—that healthful diets should be high in carbohydrate and low in fat. Unfortunately, when it comes to actual practice, most high-carbohydrate, low-fat diets look pretty much like our example of the typical American diet—a nutritional nightmare that promotes obesity, heart disease, cancer, and a host of other chronic illnesses.

Why You Can't Overeat on the Paleo Diet

Most of the foods we crave—and that make us fat if we eat enough of them—contain some combination of sugar, starch, fat, and salt in a highly concentrated form. (If you think about it, sugar, starch, fat, and salt are pretty much the recipe for *all* the foods people tend to overeat.)

In nature, a sweet taste is almost always associated with fruit. This is what drew our ancestors to strawberries, for instance—the desire for a "sweet." However, as a bonus, they got much more than the sweet taste—fiber, vitamins, minerals, phytochemicals, and other healthful substances that improved their chances of survival. Similarly, our Paleolithic ancestors sought foods with a salty taste. Salt is absolutely essential for your health—but you don't need much of it. The trace amounts of salt found in fresh fruits, vegetables, and lean meats were just right for our ancient ancestors—who also got a hefty dose of potassium along with the sodium. Today, almost all processed foods are grossly overloaded with salt.

Real Food versus Fake Food

Today, much of our food is also fake. What does this mean? It's created, not natural, food. See for yourself. How about a snack of dry white flour? Of course not; by itself, flour is bland and tasteless—you'd choke on it. However, if you add water, yeast, salt, vegetable oil, and sugar and then bake the result, suddenly you've got white bread. If you take this same mixture, deep-fry it in hydrogenated fats, and then glaze it with sugar, it becomes tastier still—a glazed doughnut. Or you could add bananas and walnuts to the original dough, bake it, and coat it with sugar and margarine, and you've got banana nut bread with frosting.

If you want to feel more virtuous about the whole thing, you can substitute whole-wheat flour and honey and call it "health food." But the bottom line is that none of these highly palatable food mixtures even remotely resemble the foods that nourished all human beings until very recently. In Paleolithic times, starchy foods weren't *also salty*; now we have potato chips and corn chips. Sweet foods were never *also fat*. Now we have ice cream and chocolates. Fatty foods were almost never *also starchy*. Now we have doughnuts that are not only fatty and starchy, but sugary as well.

It is extremely easy to overeat processed foods made with

starch, fats, sugars, and salt. There is always room after dinner for pie, ice cream, or chocolates. But how about another stalk of celery or another broiled chicken breast? Many overweight people can easily polish off a quart of ice cream after a full dinner. How many could—or would—eat an additional quart of steamed broccoli? The point here is that it's very difficult to overeat real foods—fruits, vegetables, and lean meats. Fruits and vegetables provide us with natural bulk and fiber to fill up our stomachs. Because they are low-glycemic, they also normalize our blood sugar and reduce our appetites. The protein in lean meats satisfies our hunger pangs rapidly and lets us know when we are full. Two skinless chicken breasts for dinner may be filling—and two more might be impossible. Can we say the same for pizza slices?

Fake foods distort our appetites, allowing us to eat more than we really need. The most insidious—doughnuts, corn chips, vanilla wafers, croissants, wheat crackers—have a terrible one-two punch: high fats plus high-glycemic carbohydrates.

Normally, purely high-fat foods allow our appetites to self-regulate. For example, you can only eat a certain amount of pure butter before your body says "Ugh" and you become full and stop eating. However, when a high-glycemic carbohydrate sneaks in along with fat, you can continue eating the fat long after you would normally be full. The carbohydrate makes the fat taste better than it would alone (particularly if some salt and sugar are added), so you eat more. But the high-glycemic carbohydrate also may fool your body into thinking that it's still hungry.

When you eat a doughnut, for example, the high-glycemic carbohydrates cause your blood insulin level to shoot up. At the same time, your blood level of a hormone called "glucagon" tends to fall. These chemical changes cause a cascade of events that may result in impaired metabolism by limiting the body's access to its two major metabolic fuels—fat and glucose. The other important result of these chemical changes is hypoglycemia—low blood sugar, which paradoxically stimulates your appetite, making you feel hungry even though you've just eaten. These high-fat, high-glycemic carbohydrate foods perpetuate a vicious cycle of being hungry and eating and never being satisfied. They cause excessive rises in your blood sugar and insulin levels and promote rapid weight gain.

High-fructose corn syrup can make this bad situation even worse. Fructose powerfully promotes insulin resistance. It's added to almost every processed food imaginable; we get most of it from soft drinks, sweets, and baked items. But it's also an ingredient in most low-fat or nonfat salad dressings—foods many of us buy in an attempt to be more responsible, to count calories, and to limit as many unwholesome ingredients as possible. The best approach is to stay away from these foods. Stick with humanity's original fare: fruits, vegetables, and lean meats.

What to Expect on the Paleo Diet

The key to the Paleo Diet is to stay with this wonderful way of eating. I can guarantee that you will immediately feel better. Your energy level will increase; you won't have to endure that late-afternoon tiredness or "blah" feeling. In the morning, you'll wake up charged and ready to greet the new day. You'll feel better with each passing day, and as the weeks go by, you'll notice that your clothes feel a bit loose. Your weight will gradually drop—week by week—until your normal, healthy body weight is restored. For some people, this may only take one or two months; for others, six months to a year; and for those with severe weight and health problems, a year or more. But the bottom line is that *it will happen.*

Many people also experience clearing of their sinuses, less stiffness of their joints in the morning, and normalization of bowel function. Indigestion, heartburn, and acid stomach are reduced and may even vanish completely within a few weeks of adopting this diet.

People with high cholesterol and abnormal blood chemistry can expect to see improvements within two weeks of starting the diet. Blood triglyceride levels will drop within days, and the good HDL cholesterol will rise rapidly as well. In addition, for most people on the Paleo Diet, total blood cholesterol and LDL cholesterol drop within the first two weeks.

The Paleo Diet is particularly helpful for people with type 2 diabetes, cardiovascular disease, high blood pressure, kidney stones, asthma, acne, and osteoporosis. There is also a significant body of evidence suggesting that the Paleo Diet may be helpful in certain autoimmune diseases such as celiac disease, dermatitis herpetiformis, rheumatoid arthritis, multiple sclerosis, and Sjögren's syndrome. It even reduces your risk of many types of cancer.

So eat well, lose weight, and be healthy with the Paleo Diet.

3

How Our Diet Went Wrong and What You Can Do about It

The blink of an eye. That's how long, in the grand scheme of human history, we have grown food and domesticated livestock. It's been only 333 generations since this change—known as the "Agricultural Revolution"—happened, and yet we have almost completely lost track of the foods our ancient ancestors ate. The so-called new foods that agriculture gave us so completely displaced the old foods that most of us are unaware that these foods were ever new. Many people assume that cereals, dairy products, salted foods, legumes, domesticated meats, and refined sugars have always been part of our diet. Not true! We need to rediscover the foods that brought our Paleolithic ancestors vibrant health, lean bodies, and freedom from chronic disease. The foods that agreed nicely with their genetic blueprints are the same foods that agree nicely with our genetic blueprints.

But what are these foods? How can we possibly know what our Paleolithic ancestors ate? My research team and I have been asking these same questions for the past decade. I am happy to tell you that we have found answers to these questions by carefully piecing together information from four sources:

- The fossil record
- Contemporary hunter-gatherer diets

- Chimpanzee diets
- Nutrients in wild animals and plants

The Paleolithic (Old Stone Age) era began some 2.5 million years ago in Africa when the first crude stone tools were developed. It ended about 10,000 years ago in the Middle East, with the first ancient farms. (Perhaps twenty different species of ancient humans lived in the Paleolithic era. However, for the purposes of this book, we'll cover only the diets of our direct ancestors.) We can trace the evidence showing the dominance of lean meat in human diets from our origins 2.5 million years ago until the beginnings of agriculture 10,000 years ago.

Lean Meat Is Brain Food

The notion that human beings were meant to be vegetarians runs contrary to every shred of evolutionary evidence from the fossil and anthropological record. We owe a huge debt to lean meat. In fact, scientific evidence overwhelmingly suggests that if our ancient ancestors had eaten a meatless diet, we wouldn't be where we are today. I wouldn't have become a scientist, you wouldn't be reading this book, and we would all look a lot more like our nearest animal relative—the chimpanzee.

How can this be? Chimps are hairy, and they have a big gut. They swing from trees. Well, yes, but about 5 to 7 million years ago, so did our prehuman ancestors. The evidence is that the family tree forks—and humans moved into a category all their own. But genetically speaking, we are only about 1.7 percent different from the chimp.

Chimps are mostly vegetarians (although they do eat a few insects, bird eggs, and the occasional small animal), and they have the big, protruding belly characteristic of vegetarian animals (horses and cows, for example, have big bellies, too). Apes need large, active guts to extract the nutrients from their fiber-filled, plant-based diet.

About 2.5 million years ago, our ancestors began trading in their big guts for bigger brains—to the point where today our bellies are about 40 percent smaller than those of chimps and our brains are about three times larger. The turning point came when our ancestors figured out that eating animal food (meat and organs) gave them much more energy. Over the years, their bellies began to shrink—because they didn't need the extra room to process all that roughage. All the energy formerly needed by the gut was diverted to the brain, which doubled and then tripled in size. Without nutrient-dense animal foods in the diet, the large brains that make us human never would have had the chance to develop. Meat and animal foods literally shaped our genome.

Interestingly, just before the same period when human brains began to expand, something new came on the scene: tools—crude stone weapons, and knives that our ancestors used to butcher animal carcasses and later to hunt. We know this because of telltale cut marks that have been found on the bones of fossilized animals and from evidence (a classic example is the 125,000-year-old spear crafted from a yew tree found embedded between the ribs of an extinct straight-tusked elephant in Germany) compiled at thousands of archaeological sites worldwide.

At first, humans were not terribly good hunters. They started out as scavengers who trailed behind predators such as lions and ate the leftovers remaining on abandoned carcasses. The pickings were slim; ravenous lions don't leave much behind, except for bones. But with their handy tools (stone anvils and hammers), our early ancestors could crack the skulls and bones and still find something to eat—brains and fatty marrow.

Marrow fat was the main concentrated energy source that enabled the early human gut to shrink, while the scavenged brains contained a specific type of omega 3 fat called "docosahexaenoic acid" (DHA), which allowed the brain to expand. Docosahexaenoic acid is the building block of our brain tissue.

Without a dietary source of DHA, the huge expansion of our brain capacity could never have happened. Without meat, marrow, and brains, our human ancestors never would have been able to walk out of tropical Africa and colonize the colder areas of the world. If these people had depended on finding plant foods in cold Europe, they would have starved. In a landmark series of studies, my colleague Mike Richards, at Oxford University, studied the bones of Paleolithic people who lived in England some 12,000 years ago. Their diet, Richards confirmed, was almost identical to that of top-level carnivores, such as wolves and bears.

Hunting Big Game

Why would any sane person get close enough to poke a spear into a sharp-hoofed, kicking, and snorting 600-pound horse—much less a raging 5-ton mammoth? Why didn't Paleolithic people play it safe, gathering berries and nuts and snaring rabbits, rodents, and small birds? Again, the wisdom of the old ways becomes clear.

The basic idea of foraging for food—whether you're a human, a wolf, or even a house cat chasing a mouse—is simple. You've got to receive more energy from the food you capture than you use in trying to capture it. If you run around all day and use up 1,000 calories, but come home with only ten apples worth a grand total of 800 calories, you're going to be very hungry. So when Paleolithic people went looking for food, they tried to get the most bang for the buck. The best way to do this, they found, was with a large animal. It takes a lot more energy to run down and capture 1,600 one-ounce mice than it does to kill a single deer weighing 100 pounds (1,600 ounces). But there's a much more important reason why larger animals were preferred. It's called "protein toxicity."

We can only tolerate a certain amount of protein at a time—about 200 to 300 grams a day. Too much protein makes us nauseated, causes diarrhea, and eventually can kill us. This is why our Paleolithic ancestors couldn't just eat lean muscle meat. They needed to eat fat along with the lean meat, or they needed to supplement the lean meat with carbohydrates from plant foods. Early explorers and frontiersmen in North America knew this, too. They were painfully aware of the toxic effect of too much lean protein; they called the illness "rabbit starvation."

On average, large animals like deer and cows (or, for Paleolithic people, mammoths and wild horses) contain more fat and less protein than smaller animals like rabbits and squirrels. The squirrel's body is 83 percent protein and 17 percent fat; the mule deer's body is 40 percent protein and 60 percent fat. If you ate nothing but squirrel, you would rapidly exceed the body's protein ceiling, and like those early pioneers, you'd end up with rabbit starvation. On the other hand, if you only had deer to eat, you'd be doing fine. You would not develop protein toxicity because you'd be protected by the deer's higher fat content. This is why Paleolithic hunters risked their lives hunting larger animals.

In the Paleo Diet, you're protected from protein toxicity, too—by unlimited access to fresh fruits and vegetables. You're also protected by the good cholesterol–lowering monounsaturated fats and by our most powerful deterrent to heart disease—omega 3 fatty acids. With these safeguards in place, protein is your friend. High levels of protein speed up your metabolism, reduce your appetite, and lower your cholesterol. You will benefit from eating lean protein at every meal. I can assure you that as long as you eat plenty of fresh fruits and vegetables, there is no such thing as too much protein.

Restoring the Balance in Your Diet

My research team and I have found that, ideally, a little more than half—55 percent—of your calories should come from lean meats, organ meats, fish, and seafood. The balance should come from fresh fruits and vegetables, some nuts, and healthful oils.

In the average American diet, not only is the balance of plant to animal food off-kilter, it's almost exactly the opposite of what we are genetically programmed to eat. In the typical American diet, 24 percent of the calories come from cereals, 11 percent from dairy products, 18 percent from refined sugars, and 18 percent from refined oils. These foods represent 71 percent of the energy consumed in the typical American diet—yet virtually none of them are to be found on the Paleo menu of lean meats, fresh fruits, and vegetables. In the American diet, about 38 percent of the calories come from animal foods, most of them high-fat and unhealthy meats (hot dogs, fatty ground beef, bacon, lunch meats, etc.)—a far cry from the Paleo Diet.

How "Progress" Has Hurt Us

The Agricultural Revolution changed the world and allowed civilization—cities, culture, technological and medical achievements, and scientific knowledge—to develop. These were all good things. And yet, there was a huge downside. The Agricultural Revolution is also responsible for much of today's obesity and chronic disease. The foods that agriculture brought us—cereals, dairy products, fatty meats, salted foods, and refined sugars and oils—proved disastrous for our Paleolithic bodies.

Nobody could have anticipated this revolution or its consequences. The early farmers didn't have some great plan to overthrow the old system. They were just looking for better ways to feed their families in the face of a rising population and dwindling food resources. It all started in the Middle East about 10,000 years ago, when some enterprising people started to sow and harvest wild wheat seeds. Later, they domesticated barley and a few legumes and then livestock—sheep, goats, and pigs. They still picked wild fruits and vegetables and still hunted wild game, but the die was cast; the diet had changed dramatically.

Hello Grains, Hello Health Problems

The archaeological record clearly shows that whenever and wherever ancient humans sowed seeds (and replaced the old animal-dominated diets), part of the harvest included health problems. One physical ramification of the new diet was immediately obvious: early farmers were markedly shorter than their ancestors. In Turkey and Greece, for example, preagricultural men stood 5 feet 9 inches tall and women 5 feet 5 inches. By 3000 B.C., the average man had shrunk to 5 feet 3 inches and the average woman to 5 feet. But getting shorter—not in itself a health problem—was the least of the changes in these early farmers. Studies of their bones and teeth have revealed that these people were basically a mess: they had more infectious diseases than their ancestors, more childhood mortality, and shorter life spans in general. They also had more osteoporosis, rickets, and other bone mineral disorders, thanks to the cereal-based diets. For the first time, humans were plagued with vitamin- and mineral-deficiency diseases—scurvy, beriberi, pellagra, vitamin A and zinc deficiencies, and iron-deficiency anemia. Instead of the well-formed, strong teeth their ancestors had, there were now cavities. Their jaws, which were formerly square and roomy, were suddenly too small for their teeth, which overlapped each other.

What had gone wrong? How could the benign practice of agriculture—harnessing nature's bounty—have caused so many health problems? We now know that although the population was soaring, the quality of life—as well as the average life span—was in a nosedive. The new staples, cereals and starches, provided calories but not the vital nutrients of the old diet—lean meats, fruits, and vegetables. The result—ill health and disease.

The health picture got worse over the years with the arrival of salt, fatty cheeses, and butter. Our ancestors learned to ferment grains, make beer, and eventually distill spirits. Selective breeding—and the innovation of feeding grain to livestock—steadily produced fatter pigs, cows, and sheep. Most meat wasn't eaten fresh—fewer people hunted—but instead was pickled, salted, or smoked. Fruits and vegetables became luxuries—rare seasonal additions to the monotony of cereal and starch.

More recently—just 200 years ago—the Industrial Revolution brought refined sugar, canned foods, and refined white flour to the average family's table. Food was processed in earnest by the mid-twentieth century with the invention of trans-fatty acids, margarine, shortening, and combinations of these fats mixed with sugar, salt, other starches, high omega 6 vegetable oils, high-fructose corn syrup, and countless additives, preservatives, coloring agents, and emulsifiers.

Imagine a Paleolithic human confronted with a Twinkie or even a pizza. He or she wouldn't even recognize these modern-day treats as food.

Big Mistakes in the 1950s

In many ways, the 1950s were a simpler time. Part of the mind-set then seemed to be to find simple solutions for complicated problems. In the early 1950s, when scientists were unraveling the links between diet and heart disease, they found that *saturated fat* (the kind found in butter, cheese, and fatty meats) raised total blood cholesterol; it also raised the LDL (the bad kind) cholesterol level and increased the risk of heart disease. More recent research has shown that not all saturated fats raise total and LDL cholesterol. Stearic acid actually lowers blood cholesterol similar to the way that monounsaturated fats do. Unfortunately, red meat became the scapegoat; all of a sudden, it was the chief artery clogger and cause of heart attacks. Even many nutritionists and physicians jumped to the conclusion that red meat was an unhealthy food that promoted heart disease and bowel cancer.

The food industry responded to the message that saturated fats were bad by creating all sorts of "healthy alternatives"—highly polyunsaturated vegetable oils (corn, safflower, sunflower, and cottonseed, to name a few). They also gave us all kinds of products made from these oils, such as margarines, shortening, spreads, and dressings. And almost overnight, these vegetable oils and their spin-offs were incorporated into virtually all processed foods and baked goods.

Unfortunately, as we now know, this was a very bad move. The indiscriminate infusion of vegetable oils into the American diet gave us far too many omega 6 polyunsaturated fats at the expense of the good omega 3 polyunsaturated fats. And the increased use of margarine and spreads caused the widespread introduction of still another kind of fat, called "trans-fatty acids," into our meals and snacks.

The next plan the nutritional masterminds came up with—like the anti–red meat campaign, it was not well thought out and was inadequately tested before being put into practice—was to replace saturated fats with carbohydrates, primarily starchy carbohydrates, like those found in bread, potatoes, and cereals. By the early 1990s, this recommendation had become so entrenched that it was the official policy of the USDA. The bedrock of our national Food Pyramid is its base—six to eleven servings of cereal grains. We now know, from scientific studies examining something called the "glycemic index" of certain foods, that this is six to eleven servings too many.

Part of the confusion here is that all carbohydrates are not created equal. Some of them are good for us. But others promote ill health and disease, and this brings us to the glycemic index. Good carbohydrates have a low glycemic index. This means they cause a minimal or slow rise in our blood glucose (sugar) level. The "glycemic load" is the glycemic index of a food times its carbohydrate content. It is this high-glycemic load that elevates blood insulin levels in many people. High-glycemic carbohydrates cause large and rapid rises in blood glucose and have been implicated in a wide variety of chronic diseases—adult-onset diabetes, high blood pressure, heart disease, obesity, elevated blood uric acid levels, elevated blood triglycerides (the building blocks of fat, which float around in the bloodstream), elevated small-dense LDL cholesterol, and reduced HDL cholesterol. This cluster of diseases is known to cardiologists as metabolic syndrome. Regrettably, the architects of the Food Pyramid did not distinguish between high- and low-glycemic carbohydrates when they started this carbo-mania.

Let's see how our modern way of eating has deviated from the Seven Keys to nutrition I laid out in chapter 2, and how this has affected our health.

The Seven Major Problems
in the Typical American Diet

1. Not Enough Protein

Protein makes up 15 percent of the calories that most Americans (and people in other Western countries) eat every day. But it should be much higher—between 19 and 35 percent—to give us more energy and help us burn off extra calories. Look at the numbers: For every 100 calories, cereals average only about 12 percent protein—compared to 83 percent protein for game meats. Legumes like lentils, peas, and beans average 27 percent protein.

As for dairy products, the phenomenon of the "milk cow" (or goat or sheep) happened roughly 9,000 years ago. Milk contains 21 percent protein, cheese averages 28 percent protein, and butter has absolutely no protein—but a lot of fat.

The bottom line: Most of us are getting only half of the protein we need. Why is this bad? As I'll discuss in the next three chapters, a low protein intake contributes to weight gain and a high blood cholesterol level and increases your risk of many chronic diseases.

2. Too Much of the Wrong Carbohydrates

The USDA Food Pyramid is based on carbohydrates; we're a nation of starch and sugar eaters. Carbohydrates make up about half of the typical Western diet—a considerable difference from the Paleo Diet. For our ancient ancestors, carbohydrates accounted for 22 to 40 percent of the daily calories—but these were good carbohydrates, from wild fruits and vegetables. These low-glycemic foods—which don't cause blood sugar to spike—are digested and absorbed slowly.

With nonstarchy fruits and vegetables, it's very hard to get more than about 35 percent of your calories as carbohydrates. For example: There are 26 calories in the average tomato. To get 35 percent of your daily calories as carbohydrates from tomatoes only, you'd have to eat thirty tomatoes. And this is why, with the Paleo Diet, you can indulge yourself by eating all the nonstarchy fruits and vegetables you want. When you eat the right foods, getting too many carbohydrates—or eating too many high-glycemic carbohydrates, which can cause a dangerous rise in your blood sugar and insulin levels—is simply not something you have to worry about.

The average carbohydrate content of fruits is only about 13 percent per 100 grams, about 4 percent for nonstarchy vegetables—and zero for lean meats, fish, and seafood. In stark contrast, the average carbohydrate content of cereal grains is 72 percent per 100 grams.

Why are many carbohydrates bad? Many whole grains and legumes don't have a lot of vitamins and minerals. They're poor dietary sources of these important nutrients. So a diet that's tilted too heavily toward grains and legumes—at the expense of lean meats, fruits, and vegetables—can lead to vitamin and mineral deficiencies. This is why so many of our breads and cereals are fortified with extra nutrients. Food shouldn't need to be supplemented with vitamins, and if you're getting the right balance of lean meats, fruits, and vegetables, neither should you.

Worse, cereal grains and legumes even contain "antinutrients"—chemicals that actually *prevent* your body from absorbing the proper nutrients and can damage the gastrointestinal and immune systems. Too many grains and legumes can disrupt the acid balance in the kidneys as well, and can contribute to the loss of muscle mass and bone mineral content with aging.

Finally, if you eat more carbohydrates, you're eating less protein. Protein is the dieter's friend: it reduces your appetite and increases your metabolism—and this translates rapidly into weight loss.

One of the great dietary myths in the Western world is that whole grains and legumes are healthful. The truth is that these foods are marginal at best. But what about the "health-food" breads? At best, they're *less bad* than the overprocessed, super-refined white breads you could be buying. But they're still not part of the Paleo Diet. Formerly (before "progress" brought refined milling technology to bread making), almost all cereal grains either were eaten whole or were so crudely milled that nearly the entire grain—bran, germ, and fiber—remained intact, and flour was much less refined than the kind we buy today. Our great-great-grandparents ate cracked wheat breads and baked goods with a moderate glycemic index—which meant a more moderate rise in blood sugar level.

Does this mean that whole grains are good for you? Not necessarily. It just means that an extra bad characteristic—a high glycemic index—wasn't incorporated into them yet. That unfortunate addition happened about 130 years ago, when steel roller mills came on the flour-making scene. They smashed all the fiber out of the grains and left the wimpy white, high-glycemic powder most of us think of as flour. Today, almost all baked goods made with this stuff frequently cause the blood sugar level to rise excessively.

Even "whole wheat" bread made from flour ground by these steel roller mills does the same thing to your blood sugar, because the flour particle size is uniformly small—so it's virtually no different from white flour. About 80 percent of all the

> Cereal grains are literally best left for the birds

cereal products Americans eat—as they follow the directions of the USDA Food Pyramid—come from refined white flour with a high glycemic index.

Compounding the Problem: Sugar and Sweeteners

Our Paleolithic ancestors loved honey. But it was a rare treat, because it was only available seasonally and in limited quantities (and they had to outmaneuver bees to get it). So for the most part, refined sugars—another source of carbohydrates—simply were not part of humanity's diet for 2.5 million years. In fact, until about the last 200 years or so, they weren't part of anybody's diet.

Sugar is another of those side effects of technological "progress," and its rise to prominence in our daily life has been rapid. In England in 1815, the average person used about 15 pounds of table sugar a year; in 1970, the average person used 120 pounds. How much sugar do you buy a year? Do you buy another 5-pound bag every time you go to the grocery store? You're not alone.

Yet sugar, like refined cereal grains, is not good for us. Sure, it causes cavities—most of us hear that message every time we go to the dentist. But it's also becoming evident that sugar poses more serious health problems. It promotes insulin resistance and metabolic syndrome diseases almost as much as high-glycemic breads and starchy potatoes do.

The chemical name for table sugar is "sucrose." Although sucrose has nearly the same high glycemic index (65) as white bread (70), it has two additional characteristics that make it particularly harmful for insulin metabolism. First, it is 100 percent carbohydrate, meaning that its glycemic load is very high.

Second, when your body digests sucrose, it is broken down into two simple sugars—high-glycemic glucose (with a glycemic index

of 97) and low-glycemic fructose (with a glycemic index of 23). Scientists used to think that fructose was not harmful because of its
low glycemic index. But recent laboratory studies by Dr. Mike

Pagliassotti and colleagues at Arizona
State University have revealed that
fructose is actually the main culprit in
table sugar that causes insulin resistance. Dr. Pagliassotti's findings were
bolstered by research at the University of Lausanne Medical School in
Switzerland, by Dr. Luc Tappy and

To calculate the glycemic
load, multiply the
glycemic index by the
carbohydrate content

colleagues, showing that fructose can cause insulin resistance in
humans. Insulin resistance, in turn, often promotes obesity and
chronic metabolic syndrome diseases, including hypertension,
heart disease, and diabetes.

High-Fructose Corn Syrup: A Really Bad Idea

The steady increase in table sugar use was an unfortunate development in the carbohydrate content of our diet. But in the 1970s,
the food-processing industry made a discovery: high-fructose corn
syrup could save them a lot of money. Because fructose is so much
sweeter than sucrose, less of it is needed to sweeten any processed
food. Today corn syrup is the food-processing industry's sweetener
of choice. Imagine the financial incentive here: with fructose, millions of tons of sugar are saved each year.

What does this mean to average Americans? It means we are
getting grossly disproportionate amounts of sweetener in our diets.
There are about *10 teaspoons of high-fructose corn syrup in a single
12-ounce can of soda*. The average American now eats 66 pounds of
corn syrup a year, plus 64 pounds of sucrose, and an appalling
total of 131 pounds of refined sugars. When you begin the Paleo
Diet and gradually wean yourself off processed foods, your daily
sugar intake will drastically shrink—and, better still, the sugar you
get will come from healthful fruits and vegetables.

3. Not Enough Fiber

Fiber intake began to go down the day our ancient ancestors
started harvesting cereal grains. How can this be? Don't whole
grains equal fiber? When our doctors tell us to add more fiber to
our diet, don't they mean for us to eat more oatmeal? The truth is

that calorie for calorie, whole grains can't hold a candle to fruits and vegetables. Fruits on average contain *almost twice as much* fiber as whole grains. Compared to whole grains, nonstarchy vegetables have *eight times more fiber.* Sugars have absolutely no fiber.

And yet we know that dietary fiber is absolutely essential for good health. Not having enough fiber raises our risk of developing scores of diseases and health problems. A comprehensive medical text edited by Drs. Hugh Trowell, Denis Burkitt, and Kenneth Heaton has implicated low dietary fiber in the following diseases and health problems: constipation, diverticulitis, colon cancer, appendicitis, Crohn's disease, ulcerative colitis, irritable bowel syndrome, duodenal ulcer, hiatal hernia, gastroesophageal reflux, obesity, type 2 diabetes, gallstones, high blood cholesterol, varicose veins, hemorrhoids, deep vein thrombosis, and kidney stones.

4. Too Much Fat and Too Many Bad Fats

Cut the fat! If the nutritional experts have had an overriding message over the last decades, this is it.

The thing is, this dictum is flat-out wrong. We now know that it's not *how much* fat you eat that raises your blood cholesterol levels and increases your risk of heart disease, cancer, and diabetes—it's the *kind* of fat you eat. We consume too many omega 6 polyunsaturated fats at the expense of the healthful omega 3 kind. And we get plenty of those cholesterol-raising, artery-clogging transfatty acids found in margarine, shortening, and many processed foods. Finally, we eat excessive amounts of palmitic acid, a blood cholesterol–raising saturated fat found in cheeses, baked goods, and fatty processed meats, such as hot dogs, bacon, bologna, and salami.

All of those kinds of fat are bad and need to go. But in removing all fats from our diet, we are doing more harm than good. This problem is easy to solve: With the Paleo Diet—which contains healthful fats—you will automatically reestablish the proper balance of fats in your diet. You'll also lower your blood cholesterol and reduce your risk of heart disease, cancer, and other chronic illnesses.

From our analyses of the fats in wild animals, my research team and I have found that even though ancient humans ate meat at nearly every meal, they consumed about half of the palmitic acid found in the average Western diet. (Wild game meat is low in total fat and palmitic acid and high in healthful, cholesterol-lowering monounsaturated fat and stearic acid.) They also ate lots of omega 3 polyunsaturated fats.

See Appendix 2 for a table contrasting the fats in domestic and wild meats.

The ratio of omega 6 to omega 3 fats in Paleo diets was about 2 to 1; for the average American, the ratio is much too high—about 10 to 1. Eating too many omega 6 fats instead of omega 3 fats increases your risk of heart disease and certain forms of cancer; it also aggravates inflammatory and autoimmune diseases. The lean meats, fish, fruits, vegetables, and oils found in the Paleo Diet guarantee that you will have the proper ratio of omega 6 and omega 3 fats—and of all other fats.

Cereal Doesn't Help

Cereal grains are low in fat. But the little fat they do have is unbalanced—tilted heavily toward omega 6. For example, in game and organ meat, the average ratio of omega 6 to omega 3 is 2 or 3 to one. In eight of the world's most commonly consumed cereals, this ratio is a staggering 22 to 1.

Cereal grains also have contributed to generations of blubbery cows that bear little resemblance to the lean wild animals our ancestors ate. Grain-fed cows have become loaded down with palmitic acid; worse, the fats in their meat have taken on the same high omega 6 to omega 3 ratio that's in their grain.

Milk Doesn't Help, Either

Dairy foods have taken a further toll on humanity's health over the last 9,000 years or so. Milk, cream, cheese, butter, and fermented milk products (including yogurt), ice cream, and the many processed dairy products of the twentieth century are some of the richest sources of certain saturated fats in the typical Western diet. In particular, fatty dairy foods contain palmitic and myristic fatty acids—two substances that elevate blood cholesterol. When you evaluate dairy products for fat percentage by calories, butter is the worst at 100 percent fat. Cream is 89 percent fat, cheeses average about 74 percent fat, and whole milk is about 49 percent fat. And most of the fats in these dairy products—about 40 percent—are the bad saturated fatty acids. Despite their wholesome image, whole milk and fatty dairy products are some of the least healthful foods in our diets. Their fatty acids (palmitic acid and myristic acid) raise your blood cholesterol; they also raise your risk of developing heart disease and other chronic illnesses.

The Trouble with Unbalanced Vegetable Oils

The next major misstep in food innovation happened just a few decades ago, when vegetable oils became part of our diet.

In the 1940s and 1950s, when most of these vegetable oils were introduced, nobody realized that the *ratio* of omega 6 to omega 3 fats was terribly important to health. What food scientists knew at that point was pretty simple—that polyunsaturated fats lowered blood cholesterol. And it was with this limited piece of the total picture that they happily created a great variety of cooking and salad oils that were highly polyunsaturated—but regrettably also extremely high in omega 6 fats. The worst offenders are safflower oil and peanut oil (with extremely high omega 6 to omega 3 ratios), cottonseed oil, sunflower oil, sesame oil, and corn oil. Walnut oil is more balanced. And flaxseed oil is better still—low in omega 6 fats and high in omega 3.

Trans Fats Are Terrible

Cooking and salad oils are just part of the high omega 6 problem. Nearly all processed foods—breads, cookies, cakes, crackers, chips, doughnuts, muffins, cereals, and candies—and all fast foods are cooked with some form of high omega 6 vegetable oil. Worse, many of these foods are still made with hydrogenated vegetable oils that contain harmful trans-fatty acids. Trans fats raise blood cholesterol and increase your risk of developing heart disease. A study published in the *American Journal of Public Health* concluded that consumption of trans fats by Americans was responsible for more than 30,000 deaths annually from heart disease. Trans fats are found in margarine, shortening, and some peanut butters—foods that definitely were not part of humanity's original diet.

5. Too Much Salt, Not Enough Potassium

Paleo diets were exceptionally rich in potassium and low in sodium. Just about everything Paleolithic people ate—meats, fish, fruits, vegetables, nuts, and seeds—contained about five to ten times more potassium than sodium. This means that when you eat only fresh, unprocessed food, it's impossible to consume more sodium than potassium.

We don't know exactly when farmers began to include salt in their diet, but we can guess why. Salt performed a great service, in the centuries before refrigeration, in preserving meats and other foods. It helped make foods like olives edible; it added flavor to bland cereals and other foods. At least 5,600 years ago, archaeological evidence shows us, salt was mined and traded in Europe. It remains a staple today; in fact, the average American consumes about twice as much sodium as potassium. And that's not healthy.

6. An Acid-Base Imbalance

Very few people—including nutritionists and dietitians—are aware that the acid-base content of your food can affect your health. Basically, this is what happens: everything you digest eventually reports to the kidneys as either an acid or an alkaline base. Acid-producing foods are meats, fish, grains, legumes, dairy products, and salt. Alkaline-producing foods are fruits and vegetables. You need both kinds—acid and alkaline. Fats are generally neutral.

The average American diet is slightly acidic—which means that our kidneys must handle a net acid load. For example: Suppose you have a typical "light" lunch, probably available at a dozen places near your home or office, of pepperoni pizza and a small salad with Caesar dressing. This meal is a disaster for the body's acid-base balance: the pizza's white-flour crust, melted cheeses, and salty pepperoni are all highly acidic. Add salt, and you make it even more acidic. Any alkaline remnant available in the tiny salad is neutralized by the salt and cheese in the Caesar salad dressing.

In the long run, eating too many acid foods and not enough alkaline foods can contribute to bone and muscle loss with aging. There are more immediate dangers, too: excessive dietary acid can raise blood pressure and increase your risk of developing kidney stones. It can also aggravate asthma and exercise-induced asthma.

7. Not Enough Plant Phytochemicals, Vitamins, Minerals, and Antioxidants

The Paleo Diet is rich in vitamins and minerals. One of the best ways to prove how healthy our diet used to be is to show what happened when our ancestors fiddled with it.

Vitamin C deficiency, a disease unknown to Paleolithic people, causes scurvy. Paleolithic people didn't have this problem; their diets were extremely high in vitamin C (around 500 milligrams per day) because they ate so many fresh fruits and vegetables. But even Eskimo groups—who for thousands of years have eaten virtually no plant foods for most of the year—didn't get scurvy. How can this be? They got their vitamin C from other natural sources—raw fish, seal, and caribou meat.

But as our ancestors began eating more cereal grains and fewer lean meats, fresh fruits, and vegetables, they lost much of the vitamin C in their diets. Cereal grains have no vitamin C, which is one of the body's most powerful antioxidants. Vitamin C helps lower cholesterol, reduces the risk of heart disease and cancer, boosts the immune system, and helps ward off infections and colds.

Vitamin A deficiency, like scurvy, could only have emerged after the coming of agriculture. Paleo diets were always rich in fruits and vegetables—excellent sources of beta-carotene, a nutrient that can be converted to vitamin A by the liver. (Our ancient ancestors also ate the entire carcasses of the animals they hunted and killed, including the vitamin A–rich liver.) Again, trouble happened when cereals took over and fresh fruits, vegetables, and organ meats were pushed aside. Vitamin A is essential for all of the body's mucous membranes. Vitamin A deficiency results in a condition called "xerophthalmia" (dry eyes), which can lead to blindness; in fact, this is the leading cause of blindness in children worldwide. Vitamin A deficiency also impairs the body's ability to fight infection and disease.

Vitamin B deficiency is another problem. Many people believe that whole-grain cereals are rich sources of B vitamins. They're mistaken. Compared to lean meats, fruits, and vegetables, calorie for calorie, cereals are vitamin B lightweights. Even worse, as I mentioned earlier, whole grains and legumes contain antinutrients that block the absorption of B vitamins in the intestines. For instance, antinutrients called "pyridoxine glucosides" can prevent your body from getting as much as two-thirds of the vitamin B_6 you eat. In a study of vegetarian women from Nepal, Dr. Robert Reynolds, of the USDA Human Nutrition Research Center, linked the low vitamin B_6 levels in these women to the high levels of pyridoxine glucosides in their grain- and legume-heavy diets. In contrast, the availability of vitamin B_6 in lean meats is nearly 100 percent.

Another B vitamin that's poorly absorbed when you eat whole grains is biotin. Experiments by my colleague Dr. Bruce Watkins from Purdue University have shown that wheat and other whole grains impair the body's ability to get enough biotin. Biotin deficiencies result in dry, brittle fingernails and hair. Research by Dr. Richard K. Scher and colleagues at Columbia University has shown that biotin supplements reduce fingernail brittleness and vertical "ridging" in nails. But you won't need to supplement your diet if you get enough biotin (or any other vitamin or mineral) the old-fashioned way—by eating the right foods. The availability of biotin from animal foods is almost 100 percent.

Pellagra and beriberi are two of the most devastating and widespread B vitamin deficiency diseases that have ever plagued humankind. They are caused exclusively by excessive consumption of cereals. Pellagra is a serious, often fatal, disease caused by a lack of the B vitamin niacin and the essential amino acid tryptophan. In a sad chapter of U.S. history, between 1906 and 1940 there was an epidemic of pellagra in the South. An estimated 3 million people developed it, and at least 100,000 of them died. Similar outbreaks have occurred in Europe and India, and pellagra is still common in parts of Africa.

Underlying every worldwide pellagra epidemic was excessive consumption of corn. Corn has low levels of both niacin and tryptophan, and the tiny amounts of niacin that are present are poorly absorbed. Pellagra could never have happened in the Paleolithic era, because lean meats are excellent sources of both niacin and tryptophan. Invariably, whenever we stray from the lean meats, fruits, and vegetables that we are genetically adapted to eat, ill health is the result.

Beriberi, caused by a deficiency of vitamin B_1 (thiamin), ultimately causes paralysis of the leg muscles. This disease was virtually unknown until the introduction of polished rice in the late 1800s. In parts of Japan and Southeast Asia, where rice was the staple food, beriberi became epidemic as people replaced their traditional brown rice with white rice. Eventually, scientists discovered that removing the thiamin-containing bran during the polishing process was largely responsible for this disease. Beriberi has been mostly eliminated with the introduction of "enriched" rice, to which vitamin B_1 is added. However, the message should be clear: If we have to add a vitamin to a food to prevent it from causing ill health and disease, we shouldn't be eating it in the first place.

Vitamin B Deficiency and Heart Disease

In North America, we enrich our refined cereal grains with vitamin B_1 and niacin—which means you will never have to worry about pellagra or beriberi. But it doesn't mean that these foods are good for you. Far from it. Within the past twenty years, a major risk factor for heart disease has surfaced. It has been found that low dietary intakes of three B vitamins—B_6, B_{12}, and folate—increase your blood level of an amino acid called homocysteine. A high blood level of homocysteine, in turn, increases your risk of heart disease. Whole-grain cereals have no vitamin B_{12}, their vitamin B_6 is poorly absorbed, and they are at best a meager source of folate. So excessive consumption of whole-grain cereals instead of lean meats, fruits, and vegetables is a formula for disaster for your heart. Again, lean meats are rich sources of vitamins B_6 and B_{12}, and fresh fruits and vegetables are our best food sources of folate. By eating the foods nature intended, you will never have to worry about your B vitamin status, homocysteine level, and heart disease.

Folate Deficiency

Since most Americans don't eat enough fresh fruits and vegetables, our dietary intake of folate is often marginal or low. Folate not only protects us from heart disease, it reduces our risk of colon cancer. Taken by pregnant women, it prevents spina bifida. Because of these healthful effects, the U.S. government now enriches our refined cereal grains with folic acid (a form of folate). So, somewhat paradoxically, you can now eat white bread, doughnuts, and cookies to increase your folic acid intake—but when you eat whole grains, you won't get this benefit.

The bottom line is that grains are an inferior food. No matter how you slice your bread (whole or refined), grains are not good for you. Even when they're artificially pumped full of vitamins and minerals, they cannot measure up to lean meats, fruits, and vegetables.

Minerals

On paper, whole grains appear to be a fairly good source of many important minerals, such as iron, zinc, copper, and calcium. Actually, cereals are lousy sources of these nutritionally important minerals.

Iron

Remember the antinutrients that block our absorption of B vitamins? Other antinutrients, called "phytates," chemically bind iron, zinc, copper, and calcium within grains and block their absorption during digestion. Phytates do their job so well that the worldwide epidemic of iron-deficiency anemia—which affects 1.2 billion people—is universally attributed to the poor availability of iron in cereal- and legume-based diets. Iron-deficiency anemia weakens you and hinders your ability to work; it also makes you more susceptible to infection and more likely to develop a severe infection. It increases a mother's risk of dying during childbirth. It can permanently impair a child's learning ability. Iron-deficiency anemia—like the other deficiency diseases caused by agriculture's new foods—would not have been possible with Paleo diets. Lean meats and animal foods are rich sources of iron. More important, the type of iron found in lean meats and animal foods is easily assimilated by the body.

Zinc

Zinc deficiency is another disaster caused by whole-grain cereals. In much of the Middle East, a whole-wheat flatbread called tanok contributes more than half of the total daily calories. Studies done by Dr. John Reinhold and colleagues have shown that tanok causes a zinc deficiency that stunts growth and delays puberty in children. We need zinc to help us fight infection and colds, to sustain our strength, and to enable us to work. Once again, lean meats are excellent sources of zinc. In fact, the "bioavailability" (the amount you receive of a particular nutrient) of zinc from meat is four times greater than from grains.

Calcium

Most American women, and many men, have gotten the message about calcium: insufficient dietary calcium can eventually lead to bone loss and osteoporosis. Few realize that cereal grains and legumes are a catastrophe for your bone health. As with iron and zinc, the little calcium that's present in whole grains is bound to phytates—which means that most of it never gets absorbed by the body. Cereals also contain high levels of phosphorus. We know that an unfavorable calcium-to-phosphorus ratio can speed up bone loss. Also, cereals produce a net acid load to the kidneys— and this, too, increases calcium loss in the urine.

Whole grains are even known to disrupt vitamin D metabolism in the body. Vitamin D increases calcium absorption and prevents rickets, a disease that causes bone deformities. In fact, scientists who want to study rickets in laboratory animals know exactly how to produce it—by feeding the animals whole grains. In many of the world's undeveloped countries, where whole grains and legumes are the main sources of calories, rickets, osteoporosis, and other bone-mineral diseases are common.

From the fossil record, we know that these same bone-mineral problems were also common among the first farmers. Not surprisingly, the hunter-gatherers who came before them didn't have these diseases. Hunter-gatherers never drank milk. They did not have bone-mineral problems because they ate lots of fruits and vegetables—which gave them enough calcium to build strong bones. Fruits and veggies also gave them an abundant source of alkaline base that prevented excessive losses of calcium in the urine. When you adopt the Paleo Diet, you won't have to worry about your calcium intake. You'll get all you need from the fruits and vegetables. But more important, you'll be in calcium balance. You will be taking in more calcium than you lose, and this is essential for bone health.

By restoring lean meats, fruits, and veggies to your diet and eliminating agriculture's new foods, you will lose weight, feel better, and reduce your risk of developing the diseases of civilization that plague us all.

PART TWO

Losing Weight and Preventing and Healing Diseases

4

Losing Weight the Paleo Diet Way

Here are four reasons why you should make lean protein a major part of your diet:

- It can't be overeaten.
- It raises your metabolism, causing you to burn more calories.
- It satisfies your appetite, causing you to feel less hungry between meals.
- It improves insulin sensitivity.

Determining Whether You Need to Lose Weight

How do you know if you're overweight? Scientists have devised a simple measure based on your height and weight that allows you to know exactly how much extra weight you may be toting. This measure system is called the "body mass index" (BMI), and here are the categories:

BMI	Classification
Below 18.5	Underweight
18.5–24.9	Normal
25.0–29.9	Overweight
Above 30.0	Obesity

The BMI is easy to calculate. It is simply your weight in kilograms (kg) divided by your height in meters (m) squared. You can calculate your weight in kilograms by dividing your weight in pounds by 2.2. You can change your height to meters by multiplying your height in inches by 0.0254. So a 5-foot, 4-inch (64 inches) tall woman who weighs 154 pounds would weigh 70 kilograms (154 / 2.2 = 70 kg), and her height in meters would be 1.63 meters (64 × 0.0254 = 1.63 m). Her height in square meters would be 2.66 (1.63 × 1.63 = 2.66). Her BMI would be 26.3 (70 / 2.66 = 26.3). This would put her in the overweight category. If your BMI is greater than 27, this may be a sign that you are insulin resistant and have (or are at high risk of developing) one or more of the diseases of metabolic syndrome.

A Doctor Loses 30 Pounds: Ben's Story

Here is what Dr. Ben Balzer, a general family physician from Sydney, Australia, has to say about the Paleo Diet:

> In April this year, I reached the end of my tether with my weight. I'd tipped the scales at 222 lbs. My weight for my height should be under 172 pounds. In fact, I'd been too frightened to get on the scales for some weeks, as I knew what they would tell me. I'm sure I hit 225 pounds during this time. I'd been following the standard dietary advice of low-fat dieting reasonably well for seven years. Although it worked well at first, it stopped, and my weight had gradually increased.
>
> As a doctor, I knew exactly what I was in for. I have a strong family history of diabetes, hypertension, stroke. I was 37 years old. Medically, I knew it was inevitable that I would be affected if I didn't act. I was feeling tired, bloated, and sluggish. It seemed harder to get through each day. I tried to exercise but had trouble finding the time and could swim only 500 meters with difficulty. My feet were also hurting badly. I had had heel pain syndrome (heel spur) for two and a half years, despite cortisone shots and physical therapy. I had headaches at least five days a week.
>
> Fortunately, 10 years earlier I'd heard a noted Australian professor of medicine mention the Paleolithic diet. That sounds like a logical idea, I thought, and filed it away for future reference; there was no Internet then. In my time of need, I searched the Internet for Paleolithic diet and immediately found Don Wiss's

www.Paleofood.com site. Also, a local dietitian recommended a scientific paper by Eaton, Eaton, and Konner, and I was off.

The first thing that I noticed on the diet was a feeling of a surge in my vitality. Within two weeks, my heel pain syndrome disappeared—a totally unexpected effect. My headaches soon reduced to once each two weeks and after eight months are down to once each 6 weeks or so and very mild at that—another unexpected effect.

The weight fell off very quickly—15 pounds in the first month, and now 29 pounds altogether. If that wasn't enough, I've had an increase in my muscle bulk, despite having little chance to exercise. The end result was that my trousers were almost falling off me, but my shirts were getting tight across the shoulders. The effect on my fitness was immediate. The first time I went swimming on the diet, I clocked up 1,000 meters and was hardly puffing afterward. I can run around better than I can ever remember.

My mental clarity has improved and is sharper than it has ever been before in my life. Everyone who knows me tells me how well I look. Interestingly, when I socialize, I'll often break the diet to be sociable. If I eat bread twice on the one weekend, I'll always get up on the Monday morning with sore heels again.

Since then, I've studied the diet intensively. I am totally convinced [that] far more illnesses than [were] previously suspected are related to factors in the modern diet. In addition to the usual illnesses listed as dietary (hypertension, diabetes, hypercholesterolemia, cardiovascular disease, stroke), we can add many forms of arthritis, throat infection, peptic ulcer, acne, and many others.

I plan to stay on the Paleolithic diet (as well as one can in this modern age) for the rest of my life. I think it's obvious from the above that I would be silly if I didn't!

A lean and healthy body is your birthright. The Paleo Diet is not a quick-fix solution. It is not a temporary, gimmicky diet. It's a way of eating that will gradually normalize your body weight to its ideal level and keep the pounds off permanently.

There's one very simple concept that you must understand when it comes to losing weight—the First Law of Thermodynamics, which states that energy is neither created nor destroyed. This means that the energy—calories—you put into your body must equal the energy you expend. Otherwise, you'll either gain or lose weight. If you eat more calories than you burn off, you'll gain weight. If you burn more than you take in, you'll lose weight.

Why Protein Helps Burn Calories

When it comes to human metabolism, this basic law of physics is a bit more complicated: *All calories are not created equal.* Protein is different from carbohydrates and fats.

How do you burn calories? Some you burn at a very low level all the time as part of your "resting metabolism"—for basic, unconscious functions such as beating of the heart, breathing, and digestion. You burn more calories when you move and still more when you exercise.

The common wisdom is that there are only two ways to burn more calories than you eat: Eat less or move around—exercise—more.

But there's another way to burn calories—a subtle process that can work wonders over weeks and months to create a substantial, long-term caloric deficit. Best of all, you don't even have to get out of bed to reap the benefits. This amazing phenomenon is called the "thermic effect," and the key to making it work is protein.

This is how it works: During the digestive process, your body breaks down food into its basic components—carbohydrates, fats, and proteins—and turns them into energy it can use. There's a trade-off: To get the energy from the food, the body must spend some of its own energy. There's a scientific name for this use of energy to digest and metabolize food—"dietary-induced thermogenesis" (DIT). Carbohydrates and fats generate about the same low DIT. Protein's DIT is huge in comparison—more than two and a half to three times greater. So, in order for the body to obtain energy from dietary protein, it must give up almost three times more energy than it needs for either fat or carbohydrates.

What this means is that *protein boosts your metabolism and causes you to lose weight* more rapidly than the same caloric amounts of fat or carbohydrates. A study carried out at the Dunn Clinical Nutrition Center in Cambridge, England, by Dr. M. J. Dauncey and col-

---

Over six months—with absolutely no increase in exercise or decrease in caloric intake—a high-protein diet could cause you to lose **10** to **15** pounds. Over those same six months—with increased exercise and a somewhat decreased caloric intake—a high-protein diet could cause you to lose **30** to **75** pounds!

leagues showed that during a twenty-four-hour period, a high-protein diet increased total energy expenditures by 12 percent (220 calories) compared to a calorically matched high-carbohydrate diet.

Think about it. You don't have to cut calories one bit. You can lose 20 to 30 pounds in a year with utterly no change in the quantity of food you eat or even any change in your exercise habits. Or a lot more than that if you exercise more or eat less. That's just what happened with Dean.

Losing 75 Pounds in Six Months: Dean's Story

In April 1999, *Dateline NBC* ran a feature story of my research into Paleo diets and interviewed Dean Stankovic, age thirty-two. Dean's weight had fluctuated wildly on his 6-foot, 3-inch frame since his graduation from high school, at one point reaching a high of 280 pounds. Before he adopted the Paleo Diet, Dean had tried dozens of diets. Although Dean was very determined to lose weight, he just couldn't seem to stick to traditional low-calorie diets like the one created by Weight Watchers. They made him feel hungry all the time. Worse, on all of these diets, his weight dropped at first—but the longer he stayed with them, the slower the weight loss became. This is because the body's metabolic rate slows down to conserve body stores during periods of starvation—which is exactly what low-calorie diets are. Eventually, after a few months of starvation with these low-calorie diets, no matter how strong his willpower and resolve, Dean always went back to his normal way of eating—basically, the standard American diet.

Dean had tried the high-fat, low-carbohydrate diets advocated by Dr. Atkins and others. He lost weight with these diets but complained of a low energy level, lethargy, and constant fatigue. He also believed that all of those fatty, salty, bacon-and-egg breakfasts, greasy sausages and salami, and fatty cheeses just couldn't be good for his body. And these diets became boring. It was fun at first to trade in one evil (sweets and starches) for another (fats). But after a while he craved apples, peaches, and strawberries—any fresh fruit. Dean just couldn't imagine going through the rest of his life eating only tiny amounts of fruits and veggies. This was not a lifelong way of eating! Life was not worth living when all he had to look forward to was fatty meats and cheeses, cream, and butter. Dean's mind and body rebelled, and he found himself once again down in the dumps—back to his old diet and back to his old weight.

In the fall of 1998, Dean met a young woman who had been eating in the Paleo manner for a number of years. She gave Dean some of my writings and dietary recommendations. After a few false starts, Dean began the Paleo Diet in earnest and started to lose weight steadily. By the spring of 1999, after six months on the Paleo Diet, he had lost 70 pounds and was down to a svelte 185 pounds. Dean's opening remark on *Dateline NBC*—"It is a very satisfying diet; I don't feel hungry"—is a characteristic comment, echoed by almost everyone who gives this way of eating a try. Two years later, Dean has kept the weight off and sums up his feelings this way: "I consider it more than just a diet; it's more of a lifestyle. I think it is one of the greatest diets ever created. I have no plans to go back to my old ways."

Protein Satisfies Your Appetite

Protein's high DIT is not the only reason you lose weight when you start eating more lean animal protein. Protein also affects your appetite. Protein satisfies hunger far more effectively than either carbohydrate or fat. Dr. Marisa Porrini's research group at the University of Milan in Italy has found that high-protein meals are much more effective than high-fat meals in satisfying the appetite.

High-protein meats also do a much better job of reducing hunger *between meals* than do high-carbohydrate vegetarian meals. Dr. Britta Barkeling and colleagues at the Karolinska Hospital in Stockholm served twenty healthy women lunches of identical caloric value; the women ate either a high-protein meat casserole or a high-carbohydrate vegetarian casserole. The researchers then measured how much food the women ate at dinner. The women who had eaten the meat casserole ate 12 percent fewer calories during their evening meal. As this study illustrates, protein's powerful capacity to satisfy hunger not only influences how much you eat at the very next meal but also how much you'll eat all day long.

At the Rowett Research Institute in Great Britain, Dr. R. James Stubbs and colleagues fed six men a high-protein, high-fat, or high-carbohydrate meal at breakfast and then monitored their feeling of hunger for the next twenty-four hours. The high-protein breakfast suppressed hunger much more effectively than the other two breakfast meals did—even more than the high-fat breakfast. These experiments and many others have convincingly shown that if you want to feel less hungry and stay less hungry, lean animal protein is your best line of attack.

Theoretically, any leftover calories—whether they're from protein, carbohydrates, or fats—would count as a calorie "surplus" and result in weight gain. In reality, the body doesn't work that way. It is very difficult and inefficient for the body's metabolic machinery to store excess protein calories as fat. The surplus almost always comes from extra fats or carbohydrates—and these are the foods that most frequently make you fat.

It is impossible to overeat pure protein. In fact, you couldn't gain weight just on lean, low-fat protein if your life depended on it. The body has clear limits, determined by the liver's inability to handle excess dietary nitrogen (released when the body breaks down protein). For most people, this limit is about 35 percent of your normal daily caloric intake. If you exceed this limit for a prolonged stretch of time, your body will protest—with nausea, diarrhea, abrupt weight loss, and other symptoms of protein toxicity.

But remember, protein is your best ally in waging the battle of the bulge—and when it is accompanied by plenty of fruits and veggies and good fats and oils, you will never have to worry about getting too much protein. Now let's take a look at the next major reason why the Paleo Diet causes you to lose weight without nagging hunger.

Promoting Weight Loss by Improving Your Insulin Sensitivity

The Paleo Diet promotes weight loss not only because of its high protein level that simultaneously revs up your metabolism and reduces appetite, but also because it improves your insulin metabolism.

Insulin resistance is a serious problem, and most people who are overweight have it. In insulin resistance, the pancreas (the gland that makes insulin) must make extra insulin to clear blood sugar—glucose—from the bloodstream. There's a bit of a "chicken and egg" argument as to which event happens first. Does being overweight cause insulin resistance or vice versa? Scientists aren't entirely sure. However, once insulin resistance starts, it prompts a domino effect of metabolic changes that encourage weight gain. The body frequently stores more fat, for one thing. For another, excessive insulin in the bloodstream can cause low blood sugar (a condition called "hypoglycemia"). The body's response to low blood sugar is: "Hey—we're in trouble. We'd better eat something fast!" Low blood sugar stimulates the appetite, and this can be deceptive: it causes you to feel hungry even if you've just eaten.

The good news is that what you choose to eat—protein, fats, or carbohydrates—can influence the progression of insulin resistance. Dr. Gerald Reaven's research at Stanford University has shown that low-fat, high-carbohydrate foods hinder insulin metabolism. But *high-protein diets are known to improve insulin metabolism.* Dr. P. M. Piatti and colleagues at the University of Milan put twenty-five over-weight women on one of two diets. The first contained 45 percent protein, 35 percent carbohydrates, and 20 percent fat. The second contained 60 percent carbohydrates, 20 percent protein, and 20 percent fat. After twenty-one days the women on the high-protein diet had significantly improved insulin metabolism, but those on the high-carbohydrate diet actually got worse.

With all these benefits, it seems obvious that lean protein should be the starting point for all weight-loss diets. Prior to 2002, only three clinical trials of high-protein diets had been conducted. All three investigations found high-protein diets to be excellent—far better than low-fat, high-carbohydrate diets—at promoting weight loss.

Dr. Arne Astrup's nutritional research group at the Royal Veterinary and Agricultural University in Copenhagen, Denmark, studied weight loss in sixty-five people placed on either high-protein or high-carbohydrate, reduced-calorie diets. After six months, those in the high-protein group had lost an average of 19.6 pounds—and 35 percent of the participants in this group had lost more than 22 pounds. The people in the high-carbohydrate group, however, lost only an average of 11.2 pounds; only 9 per-cent of the people in this group lost 22 pounds.

Dr. Hwalla Baba and colleagues at the American University of Beirut demonstrated almost identical results when they put thir-teen overweight men on high- and low-protein, reduced-calorie diets. After only a month the average weight loss for men on the high-protein diet was 18.3 pounds compared to only 13.2 pounds for the high-carbohydrate group.

Dr. Donald Layman, a professor of nutrition at the University of Illinois, studied twenty-four overweight women who for ten weeks were on 1,700-calorie-a-day diets. Half of the women followed the current USDA Food Pyramid guidelines recommending a diet of 55 percent carbohydrate, 15 percent protein (68 grams per day), and 30 percent fat. The other half had a diet of 40 percent carbohydrate, 30 percent protein (125 grams a day), and 30 percent fat. The average weight loss for both groups was about 16 pounds, but the high-protein group lost 12.3 pounds of body fat and just 1.7 pounds of muscle compared to 10.4 pounds of body fat and 3 pounds of muscle for the Food Pyramid group. Interestingly, the study also found that women on the higher-protein diet had higher levels of thyroid hormone, which indicates that they had a faster metabolic rate. The higher-protein diet also resulted in a noticeable drop in triglyceride levels and a slight increase in the good HDL cholesterol.

In the eight years since I wrote the first edition of this book, numerous human clinical trials have conclusively demonstrated the superiority of high-protein diets in producing weight loss and benefiting overall health.

What You Can Expect to Lose on the Paleo Diet

When you start the Paleo Diet, you'll probably realize—perhaps with a shock—just how much of your diet has been built around cereal grains, legumes, dairy products, and processed foods. Even most vegetarians must eat large amounts of grains and legumes to make their plant-based diets work, because it's very difficult to get enough calories just from eating fruits and vegetables. Except for the 2,000 or fewer hunter-gatherers still remaining on the planet, none of the world's people obtain their daily sustenance just from fruits, vegetables, lean meats, and seafood. When you start the Paleo Diet, you may choose to count yourself among the dietary elite—knowing that about 6 billion people on the planet aren't eating this way. And yet just 10,000 years ago—a mere drop in the bucket of geological time—there wasn't a single person who did *not* follow the Paleo Diet.

Everything I'm telling you about how the Paleo Diet will affect your body weight, health, and well-being is based on scientifically validated information that has been published in high-quality, peer-reviewed scientific and medical journals.

If you're overweight, the Paleo Diet will normalize your weight. This means that you will steadily lose pounds, as long as you continue to follow the diet, until your weight approaches its ideal. Most people experience rapid weight loss within the first three to five days. This is mainly water loss, and it stabilizes fairly quickly. After that, how much weight you lose will depend on two things—how overweight you are to begin with and how many total "deficit" calories you accumulate. After the initial water loss, it takes a deficit of 3,500 calories to lose a pound of fat. It is not unusual for people who are obese (medically, this means people who have a body mass index (BMI) of greater than 30) to lose between 10 and 15 pounds each month.

Sharing Success Stories

Many people, in many countries, have adopted Paleo Diets to improve their health and to lose weight. You can read about their stories and triumphs at my Web address: www.thepaleodiet.com/success_stories/. You may also want to visit my blog (http://thepaleo diet.blogspot.com/), where Paleo dieters share experiences, offer support, and talk to one another about daily challenges, dietary issues, and health issues concerning the Paleo Diet lifestyle.

Losing 45 Pounds and Healing Crohn's Disease: Sally's Story

Sally is a manager for a large telecommunications company in Illinois. Her reasons for adopting the diet were primarily health-related. However, she also benefited from the diet's remarkable ability to normalize excess body weight.

> In the fall of 1986, I became severely ill. It started with several months of unshakable diarrhea, followed by gut-wrenching pain. It became so bad that I could not keep any food down. I lost 70 pounds in three months, and I was only thirteen years old. I barely made it through my classes at school, and then I'd go home and sleep. My best friends no longer came over, my mother

was sick with worry, and my father thought I was anorexic. When my symptoms began, doctors could not find anything wrong except for "perhaps some allergies." And when my symptoms grew worse, I was shuffled back and forth between doctors and specialists, each speculating on tumors, liver disease, and other life-threatening conditions. I was subjected to every conceivable test: MRI [magnetic resonance imaging], ultrasounds, upper/lower GIs [gastrointestinal studies], blood tests, stool samples, urine tests, X-rays, throat scopes, and others. It took almost nine months to reach the diagnosis of Crohn's disease.

I was given large doses of prednisone [a steroid drug] and scheduled to have a portion of my bowels surgically removed if I didn't respond to the medication. Within days of [taking] the steroids, I felt much better. Within weeks I was outside mowing the lawn and eating more in a day than I had eaten previously in a month. At the time, my medications were a miracle.

For most of my life I have been cycling between steroids, anti-inflammatory drugs, and immune suppressors. All of these medications alleviated the symptoms, but none treated the underlying disease. My overall health slowly deteriorated. I was severely depressed and powerless to stop my life from slowly wasting away. When questioning doctors, I was given unhelpful speculations: "Crohn's disease is genetic; it runs in families. It may be caused by a virus or bacterium, it is not contagious, and we do not know what causes this disease." Every specialist I saw agreed that Crohn's is not diet-related.

By the time I graduated from college, I became determined to do something. I enrolled in graduate school to learn more about scientific research so that one day I might help find a cure. While in graduate school, I discovered literature about diet-related treatments for a whole range of degenerative illnesses, including Crohn's disease. All of the diets used to treat Crohn's disease are very similar to a Paleolithic diet. It became my turn to become responsible for my own health, and I started eating a strict Paleolithic diet. The results were amazing. Within a month I was 90 percent symptom-free. I felt like I had been reborn.

I have been on the diet for almost two years now. I've lost 45 pounds and am near my optimal weight. I am 100 percent symptom-free of Crohn's disease and haven't seen a doctor in over a year. I've started running 4 miles a day, something that I could never have achieved before. This diet is anything but a quick fix. It takes time to heal the wounds of disease and medication. However, to anyone looking for control over their disease or their weight, I urge them to give it a try. It might just save your life as it saved mine.

Vegetarian Isn't Better: Ann's Story

After high school graduation, Ann Woods left her home for a summer waitressing job in Alaska. She had a great time living away from her parents and partying with her friends, but the continual stream of on-the-job glazed doughnuts, burgers, and fries, along with evening treats of M&Ms and Baskin-Robbins ice cream, eventually caused her waistline to balloon. When she came back home to start college in the fall, her weight had jumped from 110 to 135 pounds. She was still not fat but was much heavier than she had ever been. After a bit of friendly razzing from her boyfriend, she managed to lose all the weight by adopting a near-vegetarian diet that emphasized grains, potatoes, lots of starch, and very little fat or meat. At the time, this seemed a prudent thing to do. After all, this type of diet was supposed to be the healthiest.

Ann also began to jog, an activity that soon blossomed into a lifetime interest in running and fitness. Her weight stabilized, and she became lean and fit. Her blood pressure and cholesterol levels were low, but after almost seven years of running, she noticed that her energy began to wane. She was continually tired and wanted nothing more than to sleep after long runs. Ann recovered from one running-related injury only to find herself injured again within weeks. Dark circles formed underneath her eyes, and she caught colds more frequently than ever. She finally discovered that she had iron-deficiency anemia caused by her "healthful" staples of oatmeal, brown rice, beans, pasta, and low-fat yogurt.

Ann discovered the Paleo dietary principles in *The Complete Book of Alternative Nutrition,* which featured my research. It made a lot of sense to her, and she gave it a try. She replaced her former vegetarian staples with lean meat, chicken, and seafood at almost every meal. Fruits and veggies were no problem—she had eaten a lot of these before her switch. Within a week, Ann noticed that her energy level was stable throughout the day. She no longer had late-afternoon slumps. Her stamina increased, and she was less tired after her runs. After three months on the diet she dropped 5 additional pounds to her present weight of 106, her stomach was now totally flat, and her muscle tone and strength were better than ever. On top of this, her iron-deficiency anemia disappeared, and the dark circles underneath her eyes vanished.

A Nutritionist Loses 30 Pounds: Melissa's Story

Melissa Diane Smith, a nutritionist and a health journalist based in Tucson, Arizona, is the coauthor of *Syndrome X: The Complete Nutritional Program to Prevent and Reverse Insulin Resistance* and is the author of *Going Against the Grain: How Reducing and Avoiding Grains Can Revitalize Your Health*. This is her story:

> In 1986, I began a job at a health spa and naturally emphasized foods in my diet that I thought were healthy—bagels, muffins, chicken-pasta dishes, chicken-rice dishes, and turkey sandwiches. This type of diet was disastrous for me. During the next year and a half, I gained 30 pounds and developed a whole host of health problems, including a very severe flulike illness that I could not shake, which was much later diagnosed as chronic fatigue syndrome.
>
> In an effort to regain my health, I tried several popular and recommended vegetarian, macrobiotic, and high-carbohydrate diets but grew weaker and sicker on each one. I continued to experiment and eventually stumbled upon the diet that turned my health around. It was based on lean animal protein and lots of nonstarchy vegetables and was entirely free of wheat or other gluten grains, dairy, legumes, processed fats, and sugar.
>
> When I ate this way, the difference in my health was dramatic. I quickly felt more energetic, mentally focused, and less sick. I also began to effortlessly lose the excess weight I had put on. Within about six months, I lost all the weight I had gained and was back to 115 pounds—size 6 for me. It was hard to turn against established nutritional wisdom, but I kept eating this way and totally recovered from chronic fatigue syndrome. The diet was the answer to regaining my health, and it's kept me trim and healthy ever since.

Losing Weight the Right Way

With the Paleo Diet, weight loss is a continuous, deliberate decline that occurs gradually, over a period of a few to many months.

There are no quick fixes here—but then again, quick fixes don't work. Most people who try such diets are unable to stick with them over the long haul.

> The Paleo Diet is a lifelong way of eating that will normalize weight in everyone

You won't feel hungry on this diet. Protein is a great satisfier. The low-carbohydrate content of the diet combined with its low glycemic load will normalize your insulin and blood sugar levels and will also help keep you from overeating. The weight that you will lose will stay off if you just stick to the diet—all the lean meats, fish, seafood, fresh fruits, and vegetables (except starchy vegetables) you can eat.

Isn't it time to get started and give your body what it is genetically programmed to eat?

5

Metabolic Syndrome: Diseases of Civilization

It requires a very unusual mind to undertake the analysis of the obvious.

—Alfred North Whitehead

Metabolic syndrome diseases—the diseases of insulin resistance—are the main health problems of Western countries, affecting as many as half of all adults and children. There are four major metabolic syndrome diseases:

- Type 2 diabetes
- High blood pressure
- Heart disease
- Dyslipidemia (low HDL cholesterol, elevated triglycerides, and high small-dense LDL cholesterol)

Gout and blood-clotting abnormalities are usually grouped with metabolic syndrome diseases, too, and so is obesity.

When people become insulin-resistant, the pancreas must secrete more insulin than normal to clear sugar (glucose) from the bloodstream. This creates a state in which the blood insulin level is elevated all the time.

Insulin is a major hormone that affects nearly every cell in the body. A chronically high blood-insulin level is thought to be the underlying culprit in all diseases of metabolic syndrome. But these are all complicated diseases, with many contributory factors.

Some scientists believe that high-saturated-fat diets make insulin metabolism less efficient. Others, including Dr. Gerald Reaven at Stanford University, believe that high-carbohydrate diets—both low- and high-glycemic foods—are to blame. Still others single out high-glycemic carbohydrates. However, the obvious has been ignored: Most people who develop obesity and diseases of insulin resistance do it with *mixtures* of high-fat and high-glycemic carbohydrates. Some examples of these bad food combinations: Baked potato and sour cream. Bread with butter. Eggs with toast and hash browns. Pizza with cheese. Ice cream, candies, cookies, chips. These and all of the other processed foods we eat contain both a high-fat component and high-glycemic carbohydrates.

With the Paleo Diet, it doesn't matter which of these kinds of foods ultimately cause insulin resistance—because these unnatural food combinations aren't part of the picture (except as Open Meal treats). Your meals won't suffer—in fact, they'll be richer, more varied, and more delicious than ever. Instead of fatty gourmet ice cream, treat yourself to a bowl of fresh blueberries or half a cantaloupe filled with diced strawberries and walnuts. Instead of fish sticks, how about peel-and-eat shrimp or a lean grilled steak? We'll get to specific recipes and meal plans later in the book.

Healing Metabolic Syndrome: Jack's Story

Jack Challem, known worldwide as the "Nutrition Reporter," is a leading health journalist with more than twenty-five years of experience reporting on nutrition research. He is a contributing editor for *Let's Live* and *Natural Health* magazines and the coauthor of a number of popular nutrition books.

When I started writing my book *Syndrome X: The Complete Nutritional Program to Prevent and Reverse Insulin Resistance,* I was in denial about having the early stages of Syndrome X. I was 48 years old, weighed 170 pounds, had a 38-inch waist, and a fasting glucose of 111 mg/dL. I should have known better. I made a point of getting back to the very diet I advocate in my book, *Syndrome X.* I also stopped eating all pasta and virtually all bread. Basically, I was following a Paleo Diet with lean meats and a lot of veggies.

In three months I lost 20 pounds and 4 inches from my waist. My fasting blood sugar was 85 mg/dL. My blood cholesterol and triglyceride values also improved. It has been extremely easy to maintain these improvements. Eating the Paleo Diet is simple and tasty.

How Insulin Resistance Increases Your Risk of Heart Disease

High-glycemic carbohydrates cause an increase in your blood triglycerides and a decrease in your good HDL cholesterol. They also cause an increase in a special type of cholesterol in your bloodstream called "small-dense LDL cholesterol." All of these changes in blood chemistry severely increase your risk of death from heart disease.

Small-Dense LDL Cholesterol

In recent years, small-dense LDL cholesterol has emerged as one of the most potent risks for atherosclerosis, the artery-clogging process. The study of atherosclerosis has become increasingly specific. First, we had cholesterol, then HDL and LDL (good and bad) cholesterol, and now a particularly bad kind of LDL cholesterol whose small, dense particles are ideal for artery blockage.

Even if you have normal total and LDL blood cholesterol levels, you still may be at risk for developing heart disease if your small-dense LDL cholesterol level is elevated.

Although low-fat, high-carbohydrate diets may reduce total and LDL cholesterol, they are useless in lowering small-dense LDL cholesterol. In fact, they make it worse. Dr. Darlene Dreon and colleagues at the University of California-Berkeley have shown repeatedly that high-carbohydrate diets increase small-dense LDL cholesterol particles in men, women, and children. High-glycemic foods increase our blood triglycerides, which make small-dense LDL cholesterol. When we lower triglycerides—by cutting out the starch and the high-glycemic carbohydrates—we automatically lower our small-dense LDL cholesterol.

The Keys to Greater Insulin Sensitivity

The Paleo Diet improves insulin sensitivity in many ways. First, because it's humanity's original low-glycemic-carbohydrate, low-sugar diet, you won't have to worry about triglycerides, HDL cholesterol, or small-dense LDL cholesterol. All of these blood values will rapidly normalize as your insulin level becomes reduced and stabilized.

The Paleo Diet's high fiber, high protein, and omega 3 fat content all improve insulin sensitivity as well. Unlike starchy carbohydrates, protein causes only small changes in your blood levels of glucose and insulin. By itself, a single meal of pure fat doesn't change these blood levels, either. The omega 3 fats that are integral to the Paleo Diet actually *improve* insulin metabolism and cause a rapid drop in blood triglycerides. The high fiber from nonstarchy vegetables and fruits found in the Paleo Diet slows the passage of carbohydrates through your intestines; this slows blood sugar rises and ultimately also improves insulin sensitivity.

Other Diseases Related to Insulin Resistance

It's only recently that scientists have begun expanding the scope of insulin resistance. In research worldwide, this condition is being linked to many other chronic diseases and health problems. Scientists are exploring the role of insulin resistance in certain types of cancer, nearsightedness, polycystic ovary syndrome, and even acne—although in all of these, as in heart disease, many causative factors are believed to be involved. It is premature to establish a direct cause-and-effect relationship. But if these diseases ultimately do turn out to have insulin resistance as their underlying cause, you'll be protected—because the Paleo Diet contains all of the dietary elements known to stop insulin resistance.

Breast, Prostate, and Colon Cancers and Insulin Resistance

Over the last five years, scientists have discovered through a chain reaction of metabolic events that elevated levels of insulin in the bloodstream increase blood levels of a hormone called "insulin-like growth factor one" (IGF-1) and decrease another hormone called "insulinlike growth factor binding protein three" (IGFBP-3). The decrease in IGFBP-3 causes tissues to be less sensitive to one of the body's natural chemical signals (retinoic acid) that normally limits tissue growth. In addition, IGF-1, a potent hormone in all tissues, is a major regulator of growth: Increased levels of IGF-1 encourage growth, and reduced levels slow growth. Children who are below normal height have low levels of IGF-1. When IGF-1 is injected into these children, they immediately start to grow taller. As you might expect, tall children have higher levels of IGF-1. Studies of growing children by Dr. William Wong and colleagues at the Children's Nutrition Research Center in Houston found that girls who were taller and heavier and who matured earlier had higher blood levels of both insulin and IGF-1 and lower levels of IGFBP-3. Diets that cause insulin resistance—particularly, high-glycemic-carbohydrate diets—increase IGF-1 levels, lower IGFBP-3 levels, and decrease tissue sensitivity to retinoic acid. These hormonal changes, in turn, accelerate growth in developing children.

What does this have to do with adult health? It's been found that IGF-1 is a powerful stimulator of cell division—growth—in *all* cells during *all* phases of life. In fact, scientists suspect that IGF-1 may be one of the primary promoters of all unregulated and tissue growth in the body. But IGFBP-3 prevents unregulated cell growth by causing cancer cells to die naturally through a process called "apoptosis." Over the last decade, numerous scientific papers have shown a strong association between elevated levels of IGF-1, lowered levels of IGFBP-3, and breast cancer in premenopausal women, prostate cancer in men, and colorectal cancer in all adults. In animal models of many types of cancer, scientists can promote cancer by adding a key ingredient—IGF-1; conversely, adding IGFBP-3 slows cancer. Synthetic derivatives of the body's natural retinoic acid powerfully inhibit the cancer process in cell cultures. So, the whole chain of hormonal events initiated by elevated blood levels of insulin tends to promote the cancer process.

Two risk factors for breast cancer are early onset of puberty and above-average height. It is entirely possible that the same high insulin levels that elevate IGF-1 and lower IGFBP-3 (in other words, the levels that make children taller and make puberty happen sooner during childhood) also increase susceptibility to cancer during adulthood.

Many women, worried about breast cancer, have adopted vegetarian diets in an attempt to reduce their risk. Unfortunately, it may be that these grain- and starch-based diets actually increase the risk of breast cancer, because they elevate insulin—which, in turn, increases IGF-1 and lowers IGFBP-3. A large epidemiological study of Italian women, led by Dr. Silvia Franceschi, has shown that eating large amounts of pasta and refined bread raises the risk of developing both breast and colorectal cancer.

Most vegetarian diets are based on starchy grains and legumes. Sadly—despite continuing perceptions of these as healthy foods—vegetarian diets don't reduce the risk of cancer. In the largest-ever study comparing the causes of death in more than 76,000 people, it was decisively shown that there were no differences in death rates from breast, prostate, colorectal, stomach, or lung cancer between vegetarians and meat eaters.

Cancer is a complex process involving many genetic and environmental factors. It is almost certain that no single dietary element is responsible for all cancers. However, with the low-glycemic Paleo Diet, which is also high in lean protein and health-promoting fruits and vegetables, your risk of developing many types of cancer may be very much reduced.

Myopia and Insulin Resistance

Because insulin resistance changes the hormonal profile of the blood to one that facilitates tissue growth, scientists have good reason to suspect that insulin resistance lies at the root of any disease in which abnormal tissue growth occurs. One extremely common such disease is myopia—nearsightedness—which affects an estimated one-third of all Americans. Myopia results from excessive growth of the eyeball. Although the eye looks normal from the outside, inside it's too long for the eye to focus properly. Myopia typically develops during the childhood growth years and usually stabilizes by the time people reach their early twenties. New evidence that implicates insulin resistance in the childhood development of myopia may be useful in preventing nearsightedness in young children.

Eye doctors generally agree that nearsightedness results from an interaction between excessive reading and your genes. If you spent your youth with your nose in a book and if nearsightedness runs in your family, chances are good that you're now wearing glasses or contact lenses. Myopia is thought to stem from a slightly blurred image on the back of your eye (the retina) that's produced as you focus on the written page. This blurred image causes the retina to send out a hormonal signal telling the eyeball to grow longer. Experiments in laboratory animals suggest that the hormonal signal is produced by retinoic acid. Excessive reading slows the retina's production of retinoic acid, a substance that normally checks or prevents the eyeball from growing too long. Additionally, recent research shows that elevated insulin also directly contributes to the excessive growth of the eyeball. This may mean that if your children's diet prevents insulin resistance during growth and development, their risk of developing myopia may be lower.

Polycystic Ovary Syndrome

Polycystic ovary syndrome (PCOS) affects 5 to 10 percent of all North American women. Women with PCOS ovulate irregularly or not at all, and their ovaries produce high levels of male hormones such as testosterone. Women with PCOS are prone to obesity, excessive body hair, acne, high blood pressure, and type 2 diabetes. They also have a seven times greater risk of heart disease and heart attack than other women do. Almost 60 percent of all women with PCOS are insulin resistant, and most of these women have elevated levels of IGF-1. Numerous clinical studies have shown that simply changing the diet—eating foods that improve insulin metabolism—can reduce many of the symptoms of PCOS. The Paleo Diet, which normalizes insulin metabolism, can greatly help women with this problem.

Acne

For years, many dermatologists believed that diet had absolutely nothing to do with acne. But very new scientific evidence has linked insulin resistance to acne. Diets loaded with sugar, fructose, and high-glycemic carbohydrates may contribute to this problem, which can be devastating. Between 40 and 50 million American teens and adults have acne.

Some striking information to support the link between acne and diet comes from Dr. Otto Schaefer, who spent his entire professional career in the wilderness of the Canadian Far North, working with Inuit natives who literally were transferred from the Stone Age to the Space Age in a single generation during the 1950s and 1960s. Dr. Schaefer reported that in those Eskimos who ate their traditional foods, acne was absent. Only when they adopted Western foods laced with refined sugars and starches and dairy products did acne appear.

Four things happen when acne develops: First, there's accelerated growth of the skin surrounding the hair follicle (called "follicular hyperkeratosis"). Second, oil (sebum) production speeds up within the follicle. Third, the cells in the follicle abnormally stick together as they are being shed, thus plugging the follicle. And, finally, the plugged-up follicle gets infected. Until recently, dermatologists didn't know why the accelerated growth occurred, why these cells became excessively cohesive, or what caused the boost in oil production. But growing evidence suggests that elevated insulin and IGF-1 are directly responsible for the increased follicular skin growth, along with reductions in circulating blood levels of IGFBP-3. Remember that high-glycemic foods raise your blood level of IGF-1 while lowering IGFBP-3. This is why low-glycemic-load, high-protein diets are so effective in eliminating acne. They put the brakes on excessive follicular skin growth.

Besides causing increases in IGF-1 and reductions in IGFBP-3, elevated insulin levels from eating high-glycemic carbohydrates cause a rise in the male hormone testosterone. It is these increases in IGF-1 and testosterone that promote the discharge of oil. This means that insulin resistance caused by high-glycemic diets may be directly responsible for the first three steps in acne development. In the last five years, dietary intervention studies and a series of epidemiological studies from the Harvard School of Public Health have conclusively demonstrated that high-protein, low-glycemic diets like the Paleo Diet improve insulin metabolism and can help prevent acne. It is now safe to say that the Paleo Diet will improve your insulin metabolism—and if you have acne, this lifetime program of healthy eating will help it disappear.

As you can see, the Paleo Diet can be a very effective tool in fighting virtually all the diseases of metabolic syndrome.

6

Food as Medicine: How Paleo Diets Improve Health and Well-Being

We never used to be so sick. The white man's food is not good for us.

—Malaya Kulujuk, a Baffin Island Eskimo

The Diet-Disease Connection

Many of the chronic illnesses that plague the Western world—the "diseases of civilization"—can be attributed to dietary missteps. Diet and disease are obviously linked. And when we stray from the Seven Keys of the Paleo Diet, which stood firm for 2.5 million years, we not only develop metabolic syndrome diseases, but also increase our susceptibility to a host of other diseases.

How can we know whether a particular food, or the lack of it, in our diet is actually the factor responsible for a particular disease—or the absence of it? If you have a milk allergy or lactose intolerance, the cause and effect of your symptoms are probably painfully clear. But it's much harder—if not impossible—to foresee whether the pat of margarine (containing trans-fatty acids) you put on your toast yesterday morning will have anything to do with causing a heart attack forty years later.

Scientists and physicians use a variety of research procedures to determine whether diet and disease are linked, including dietary interventions, epidemiological studies, animal experiments, and cultured tissue studies. When the results of all four procedures are in agreement, it is quite likely that a certain food may cause a certain disease. However, in most cases the link between diet and disease is usually not this clear-cut; often, genetic susceptibility to disease further clouds the issue. In many of the diseases that we will be examining, the diet-disease connection has only been partially unraveled. Nonetheless, by adhering to the dietary guidelines of your Paleolithic ancestors, you will reduce your risk of developing these illnesses, and if you are currently suffering from one of these illnesses, your symptoms may improve with the Paleo Diet.

Metabolic Syndrome Diseases

I've already talked about the metabolic syndrome diseases (type 2 diabetes, heart disease, hypertension, dyslipidemia, obesity, PCOS, myopia, acne, and breast, prostate, and colon cancers) and how they are linked to elevated levels of insulin in the bloodstream. But all of these diseases also have other known contributing dietary factors. For example, salt is connected to high blood pressure—but so is a lack of fresh fruits and vegetables. Too much omega 6 fat in your diet at the expense of omega 3 fat can also cause your blood pressure to rise. Even a low protein intake has been linked to rising blood pressure.

Breast, prostate, and colon cancers are known to develop more often in people who don't eat enough fresh fruits and vegetables. Fruits and veggies hit cancer with a one-two punch: they're excellent sources of antioxidant vitamins and minerals that may impede the cancer process, and they also contain a variety of special substances called "phytochemicals," nutrients found in foods that are lethal to cancer cells. The study of most phytochemicals is fairly new; scientists are only beginning to understand how they work. But here are a few examples:

- Broccoli contains sulforaphanes, which chase cancer-causing elements out of cells.
- Broccoli is also loaded with cancer-fighting folic acid, vitamin C, beta-carotene, and a substance called "indole-3-carbinol," which helps improve the body's estrogens.

- Strawberries, tomatoes, pineapples, and green peppers contain *p*-coumaric acid and chlorogenic acid, compounds known to be powerful anticancer agents.
- Garlic and onions not only contain substances that will lower your cholesterol but are also rich sources of allylic sulfides, which seem to protect against stomach cancer.

As is the case with high blood pressure, eating too many omega 6 and too few omega 3 fats further increases your risk of developing breast, prostate, and colon cancers.

We may not know precisely how dietary factors cause each and every metabolic syndrome disease, but one thing's certain: when you adopt the Paleo Diet, you will be putting all known dietary factors on your side to prevent these illnesses.

Cardiovascular Diseases

The number one killer in the United States is cardiovascular disease. A staggering 35 percent of all deaths in this country result from heart attacks, stroke, high blood pressure, and other illnesses of the heart and blood vessels. Cardiovascular disease, like cancer, is a complex illness, and no single dietary element is solely responsible. However, once again, by following the nutritional principles of humanity's original diet, you will put the odds in your favor of not developing this deadly disease.

Good Fats Help Prevent Cardiovascular Disease

Good fats are what doctors call "cardioprotective." They protect the heart and the blood vessels from disease. With the Paleo Diet—unlike the average American diet—at least half of your fats are healthful monounsaturated fats. The other half is evenly split between saturated and polyunsaturated fats. There are no synthetic trans fats. And the crucial omega 6 to omega 3 fat ratio is about 2 to 1—which greatly reduces your risk of dying from heart disease.

Monounsaturated Fats

Monounsaturated fats reduce your overall risk of heart disease by lowering your level of total cholesterol—but not your beneficial

HDL cholesterol—in the blood. These healthful fats—found in abundance in the Paleo Diet—also help prevent LDL cholesterol from oxidizing (breaking down) and contributing to the artery-clogging process. Monounsaturated fats also may reduce your risk of breast cancer.

Omega 3 Fats

I've already talked about the beneficial effects of omega 3 fats on insulin metabolism and how they lower blood triglycerides. Omega 3 fats are also exceptionally potent agents in preventing the irregular heartbeats that can make a heart attack fatal. They help prevent blood clotting and ease tension in clogged arteries as well.

In a landmark dietary intervention study, French physicians Serg Renaud and Michel de Lorgeril evaluated the effect of a diet rich in omega 3 fats in 600 patients who had previously survived a heart attack. In this investigation, known as the Lyon Diet Heart Study, half of the patients were assigned to the American Heart Association reduced-fat diet, in which 30 percent of calories come from fat. The rest followed a 35 percent fat traditional Mediterranean diet that was rich in omega 3 and monounsaturated fats and fruits and vegetables.

The results were striking: compared to the patients who followed the American Heart Association Diet, those who were on the Mediterranean diet had a 76 percent lower risk of dying from another heart attack, a stroke, or another cardiovascular disease. This remarkable protection from heart disease can be yours, too. Like the Mediterranean diet, humankind's original diet is also high in cardioprotective omega 3 fats, fiber, monounsaturated fats, and the beneficial phytochemicals and antioxidant vitamins that are found in fruits and vegetables.

Diseases of Acid-Base Balance and Excessive Sodium

The average cereal-based, salt-laden, cheese-filled American diet—which is nearly devoid of fresh fruits and vegetables—tilts your body's acid-base balance in favor of acid. As we discussed earlier, grains, cheeses, meats, and salty foods yield a net acid load to the kidneys, while fruits and vegetables always generate an alkaline load. An overload of acid foods—at the expense of alkaline foods—can cause numerous health problems, particularly as you age and your kidneys become less adept at handling dietary acid.

Of the four major acid-producing foods, three—grains, cheeses, and salt—were eaten rarely or never by our Paleolithic ancestors. Instead, they ate huge amounts (by modern standards) of alkaline fruits and vegetables, which buffered the acid from their meat-rich diets.

Many chronic diseases prevalent in Western countries develop because of a dietary acid-base imbalance. These include:

- Osteoporosis
- High blood pressure
- Stroke
- Kidney stones
- Asthma
- Exercise-induced asthma
- Ménière's syndrome
- Stomach cancer
- Insomnia
- Air and motion sickness

The realization that such diverse problems could be linked to acid-base imbalance is fairly recent. Not so long ago, scientists connected many of these illnesses to too much sodium, or salt. But the chemical recipe for salt has two ingredients—sodium and chloride. And as I discussed earlier, it's the chloride part of salt that makes it acidic—not the sodium. Chloride may also be more to blame than sodium as a dietary cause of high blood pressure.

Osteoporosis

Earlier, I talked about salt's interplay with calcium in the body: people who eat a lot of salt excrete more calcium in their urine than do people who avoid salt. In turn, this calcium loss contributes to bone loss and osteoporosis, because the acidic chloride in salt must be buffered in the kidneys by alkaline base—and the body's largest reservoir of alkaline base is the calcium in our bones. When we eat salty potato chips or a pepperoni pizza, we are leaching calcium from our bones. When we do it over the course of a lifetime, we may well develop osteoporosis.

Asthma and Exercise-Induced Asthma

But salt is not just bad for the bones. Although it has not been shown to cause asthma or exercise-induced asthma, it can aggravate both conditions. Studies in humans and animals have shown that salt can constrict the muscles surrounding the small airways in the lung. My research team demonstrated that salt (both the sodium and the chloride components) increases the severity of exercise-induced asthma. We also showed that low-salt diets can reduce many symptoms of exercise-induced asthma.

Other Problems Caused by Salt

Maybe you don't salt your food. Good for you—but you should be aware that despite your good intentions, there's probably more salt in your diet than you think. The average American eats 10 to 12 grams of salt every day. Almost 80 percent of this comes from processed foods—even those considered healthful. Two slices of whole-wheat bread, for instance, give you 1.5 grams of salt. So automatically there's salt in any sandwich you make—even before you add salty meats like ham, salami, or bologna.

A high-salt diet increases your risk of kidney stones, stroke, and stomach cancer.

It also impairs sleep—this is one of the least-recognized benefits of low-salt diets. When you cut the salt out of your diet, you will sleep better almost immediately. Low-salt diets also have been shown to reduce motion and air sickness.

Many other foods are acidic and able to disrupt the body's acid-base balance. Every time you eat cereals, peanuts, peanut butter, bread, muffins, cheese, sandwiches, pizza, doughnuts, cookies—basically, any processed food—you are overloading your body with dietary acid. Unless you balance these foods with healthful alkaline fruits and vegetables, you will be out of acid-base balance—and at increased risk for many chronic diseases.

Potassium

Another crucial chemical balance in the body is that of potassium and sodium. Paleo diets contained about ten times as much potassium as sodium. The average American eats about five times as much sodium as potassium every day. The beauty of the Paleo Diet is that it swiftly returns your body to humanity's original high intake of potassium and low intake of sodium.

Digestive Diseases

Fiber is absolutely essential to your health—and at least thirteen illnesses can result when you don't get enough fiber in your diet. Some of the most common digestive diseases that develop when you eat the standard American diet with its overload of refined grains, sugars, dairy, and processed foods are:

- Constipation
- Varicose veins
- Hemorrhoids
- Heartburn
- Indigestion
- Appendicitis
- Diverticular disease of the colon
- Crohn's disease
- Ulcerative colitis
- Irritable bowel syndrome
- Duodenal ulcer
- Hiatal hernia
- Gallstones

The Paleo Diet is naturally high in fiber because of its abundance of fruits and vegetables—about three to five times as much fiber each day as there is in the average American diet.

Some people worry that lean meat–based diets are constipating. This is not true. Meat, fish, and seafood are not constipating at all. The famous Arctic explorer Vilhjalmur Stefansson spent years mapping and exploring the Far North at the turn of the twentieth century. During his expeditions on dogsleds, he frequently lived off the land for more than a year at a time. He and his men were entirely dependent on the all–animal food diet that could be obtained from hunting and fishing. Amazingly, he reported in his journal that men who had suffered from constipation on their former rations of flour, corn biscuits, rice, and breads were almost completely cured of their problem within a week of adopting the all-meat (high in protein, but with enough fat to avoid the risk of protein toxicity) menu of the Eskimos.

Years later, when Stefansson returned to civilization, he and another explorer were put on an all-meat diet for an entire year, under controlled hospital conditions, by the most respected scientists and physicians of the day. The clinical evaluations at the end of the year showed bowel function to be normal. Just like Stefansson and the Eskimos, you will not suffer from constipation when lean meat, fish, and seafood dominate your diet. In fact, you will find that most of your digestive problems will disappear.

Crohn's Disease and Ulcerative Colitis

As with every other disease of civilization, it is not the soluble fiber from fruits and vegetables that will reduce your digestive problems, but rather the entire diet. Dairy products, cereals, and yeast have been implicated time and again in the development of Crohn's disease, an inflammatory disease of the gastrointestinal tract. Elemental diets (special liquid formulas without dairy, cereal, or yeast proteins) are the first line of defense physicians use in treating these patients. Amazingly, almost 80 percent of patients achieve complete remission while on elemental diets with absolutely no drug therapy. But there is a big problem here: hardly anyone can stay on a liquid diet forever. What would you rather do, drink a liquid diet or eat humanity's real foods—fruits, veggies, and lean meats?

One of our most powerful therapies to calm down the inflammation of both Crohn's disease and ulcerative colitis (an inflammatory disease of the colon) is to prescribe fish oil capsules—an excellent source of omega 3 fats. Once again, we find that multiple elements in humanity's original diet complement one another to eliminate or prevent chronic illness. And it is our deviation from the three simple foods (fruits, vegetables, and lean meats) we are genetically adapted to eat that invariably causes us trouble and ill health.

Inflammatory Diseases

Omega 3 fats are powerful weapons in other wars as well. Perhaps because of their anti-inflammatory properties, they may prevent cancer from developing. They are also extremely effective in calming down virtually all inflammatory diseases—illnesses that end in "itis," such as rheumatoid arthritis, ulcerative colitis, and gingivitis. These amazingly healthful fats can even reduce symptoms of certain autoimmune diseases: the combination of supplementing your diet with omega 3 fats and eliminating grains, dairy foods, legumes, potatoes, and yeast may substantially reduce the severity of symptoms of these diseases.

Autoimmune Diseases

Autoimmune diseases such as rheumatoid arthritis, multiple sclerosis, and type 1 (juvenile) diabetes develop when the body's immune system can't tell the difference between its own tissues and those of foreign invaders. The result: the body attacks itself. The type of disease depends on the nature of the body's assault: When the immune system invades and destroys nerve tissue, multiple sclerosis and other neurological diseases develop. When the pancreas is the target, type 1 diabetes occurs. When joint tissues are attacked and destroyed, the result is rheumatoid arthritis.

All autoimmune diseases develop because of interactions between the genes and one or more environmental factors, such as a viral or bacterial infection or exposure to a certain food. No one knows exactly how viruses, bacteria, and foods can spark the disease in genetically susceptible people, but research from our laboratory increasingly implicates recently introduced Neolithic foods such as grains, legumes, dairy foods, potatoes, and other members of the nightshade family.

Many environmental agents have been suspected in the development of autoimmune diseases. But only one of these types has proved capable of causing a disease. Cereal grains—such as wheat, rye, barley, and oats—are responsible for celiac disease and dermatitis herpetiformis. In celiac disease, the immune system attacks and destroys cells in the intestine, leading to diarrhea and many nutritional problems. In dermatitis herpetiformis, the skin is attacked.

Withdrawal of all gluten-containing cereals causes complete remission of both diseases. Cereal grains, dairy products, and legumes are suspected in other autoimmune diseases, such as type 1 diabetes, multiple sclerosis, and rheumatoid arthritis. To date, no dietary intervention studies have been conducted to see whether Paleo diets—free of grains, dairy products, and legumes—can reduce the symptoms of these diseases. However, anecdotal reports from Canada show improvement in symptoms of multiple sclerosis patients following the Paleo Diet.

Lectins and Autoimmune Disease

My research group and I have published a paper in the *British Journal of Nutrition* describing our theory that dairy foods, grains, legumes, and yeast may be partly to blame for rheumatoid arthritis and other autoimmune diseases in genetically susceptible people. Legumes and grains contain substances called lectins. These substances are proteins that plants have evolved to ward off insect predators. Lectins can bind with almost any tissue in our bodies and wreak havoc—if they can enter the body, that is.

Normally, when we eat food, all proteins are broken down into basic amino acid building blocks and then absorbed in the small intestine. Lectins are different. They are not digested and broken down; instead, they attach themselves to cells in our intestines, where nutrient absorption takes place. The lectins in wheat (WGA), kidney beans (PHA), soybeans (SBA), and peanuts (PNA) are known to increase intestinal permeability and allow partially digested food proteins and remnants of resident gut bacteria to spill into the bloodstream. (Alcohol and hot chili peppers also increase intestinal permeability.) Usually, special immune cells immediately gobble up these wayward bacteria and food proteins. But lectins are cellular Trojan horses. They make the intestines easier to penetrate, and they impair the immune system's ability to fight off food and bacterial fragments that leak into the bloodstream.

Surprisingly, we have found that many common gut bacteria fragments are made up of the same molecular building blocks as those found in certain immune system proteins and in the tissues under attack by the immune system. This matchup—of gut bacteria or food protein, immune system protein, and body tissue protein—may confuse the immune system, causing it to attack the body's own tissues. A number of research groups worldwide have found that milk, grain, legume, and nightshade proteins can also trick the immune system into attacking the body's own tissues by this process of molecular mimicry.

If you have an autoimmune disease, there is no guarantee that diet will cure it or even reduce your symptoms, but there is virtually no risk, and there are many other great benefits from the Paleo Diet that will improve your health.

Psychological Disorders

One of the least known benefits of grain-free diets is their ability to improve mental well-being. My colleague Dr. Klaus Lorenz of Colorado State University has extensively studied how cereals may influence the development and progression of schizophrenia. In a wide-ranging review study, Dr. Lorenz concluded that in "populations eating little or no wheat, rye and barley, the prevalence of schizophrenia is quite low." Dr. Lorenz's analysis included the clinical studies by Dr. F. Curtis Dohan of the Eastern Pennsylvania Psychiatric Institute. In studies spanning almost twenty-five years, Dr. Dohan reported time and again that the symptoms of schizophrenia were reduced in patients on grain- and dairy-free diets but worsened when these foods were returned to the diet. Exactly why cereals may alter mood and mental well-being is not entirely clear. But several studies have shown that when wheat is digested, it contains a narcoticlike substance that may affect certain areas in the brain that influence behavior. Similar substances called "casomorphins" have been isolated from cow's milk; however, no one knows whether they can alter mood or behavior.

My colleague Joe Hibbeln at the National Institutes of Health has demonstrated that omega 3 fats may be effective in reducing depression, hostility, schizophrenia, and other mental disorders. His finding was confirmed in a four-month study of thirty manic-depressive patients by Dr. Andrew Stoll of the Brigham and Women's Hospital in Boston. Dr. Stoll used medicine's most powerful study tool, a double-blind, placebo-controlled trial, to compare the efficacy of omega 3 fats versus olive oil for treatment of manic-depressive illness. According to Dr. Stoll and his colleagues, "for nearly every outcome measure, the omega 3 fatty acid group performed better than the placebo group." This work lends credence to a number of recent studies demonstrating that the symptoms of depression are much lower in people who eat a lot of fish (an excellent source of omega 3 fats).

The Paleo Diet will also improve your mental outlook because it normalizes your insulin level. Almost everyone knows that a low blood sugar level can make you feel tired, irritable, and tense. When you normalize your insulin level with low-glycemic carbohydrates and plenty of lean protein, your blood sugar level will be more even throughout the day and so will your mood.

Vitamin-Deficiency Diseases

In the United States the common vitamin deficiency diseases (beriberi, pellagra, and rickets) were wiped out after World War II with the wide-scale fortification of our white flour and white rice with B vitamins and our milk and margarine with vitamin D. However, people living in less developed nations are not so lucky; these diseases still run rampant wherever diets are heavily based on cereals and legumes. It goes without saying that the world's primary vitamin deficiency diseases, including scurvy from a lack of vitamin C, are completely a result of agriculture's new foods. When you eat the way nature intended, you will protect yourself from all illnesses that develop from vitamin deficiencies.

Dental Cavities

Nearly all archaeological studies of Paleolithic people's teeth show them to be almost completely free of cavities. How can this be when they never brushed, gargled with mouthwash, or flossed? The answer is simple: with their diet of lean meats, fruits, and veggies, cavities simply couldn't get a foothold. Historically speaking, cavities and tooth decay didn't start until the coming of agriculture and its starchy, sugary foods. Cavities are caused when acid produced by certain bacteria eats away part of the enamel of your tooth. These bacteria can't set up shop in your teeth unless there is a constant source of sugar or starch that fuels their acid production.

We can learn a lot from our teeth because any food that does so much damage to our teeth can't be very good for the rest of our bodies, either. Refined sugars and starches are foreign substances to our Paleolithic bodies. We simply haven't had time to adapt to agriculture's new foods. We are best designed to run on the foods nature provided: lean meats, fruits, and veggies.

Alcoholism

Alcohol—and its enormous potential for abuse—was not part of the preagricultural equation. No alcoholic beverage has ever been linked to Paleolithic people, although it would have been possible to make alcoholic drinks from gathered honey (mead) or berries (wine) by natural fermentation. It wasn't until the Agricultural Revolution, with its abundance of starchy grains, that the first beers were brewed on a regular basis. Quite a bit later came wine, made from fermented grapes. (Because beer and wine are yeast fermentation by-products, they do not contain more than about 6 to 13 percent alcohol; the alcohol-producing yeast organisms die when the alcohol concentration rises above this level.) Hard liquor didn't come on the scene until about 800 A.D., with the invention of distillation.

In most Western countries, moderate consumption (five to ten drinks per week) of alcohol is not considered detrimental to health; in fact, it has been associated with a reduced risk of dying from all combined causes of death. Moderate alcohol consumption also may improve your insulin sensitivity and is associated with a reduced risk of other chronic diseases.

Does this mean you should take up drinking to improve your health? Absolutely not. You don't need alcohol to obtain the health and weight-loss benefits of the Paleo Diet. However, if you currently enjoy an occasional glass of wine, there is no need to forgo this pleasure. Consumption of alcoholic beverages a few times a week won't hurt your health, nor will it slow your weight loss. However, if you suffer from an autoimmune disease or another serious health problem, alcoholic beverages should not be part of your dietary equation.

Skin Cancers

Skin cancers come in three basic varieties:

- *Squamous cell* cancers, which form on the top layers of the skin
- *Basal cell* cancers, which form on the bottom layers of the skin
- *Melanomas*, which form within the skin's pigment-producing cells, the melanocytes

The American Cancer Society estimated that 2 million Americans would develop the first two types of skin cancer in the year 2010. These cancers grow slowly, rarely spread to other areas of the body, and are easily curable by early removal. An estimated 69,000 Americans were expected to develop melanoma in 2009. If detected early and surgically removed before they spread to other parts of the body, melanomas are highly curable, with 95 out of 100 people alive five years after diagnosis. But if melanomas spread to the rest of the body, they can be deadly; the five-year survival rate drops drastically, to 16 out of 100.

Scientists know that excessive sunlight exposure is linked to all three cancers. But this does not mean you should avoid sunlight in any amount. Here again, the experience of our hunter-gatherer ancestors proves helpful. Ironically, many studies have shown that people with high lifetime sunlight exposure (similar to that of hunter-gatherers) have lower rates of melanoma than those with low sunlight exposure. Also, indoor workers have a greater risk of developing melanoma than outdoor workers do. Even more puzzling, melanomas often arise in body areas that are infrequently or intermittently exposed to the sun. These unexpected findings have led researchers to believe that severe sunburn during childhood, or intense burns in body areas that are infrequently or intermittently exposed to the sun, may be more important in the development of melanoma than cumulative exposure during adulthood.

When your exposure to sunlight is gradual, moderate, and continuous—if you don't get excessive sunburn—your body responds in a manner guided by evolutionary wisdom. The skin begins to tan from increased production of melanin, and the darkened skin provides protection from the sunlight's damaging ultraviolet rays. Also, vitamin D levels in the blood begin to rise as ultraviolet light strikes the skin, causing it to convert cholesterol into vitamin D.

Vitamin D is a potent inhibitor of the cancer-causing process. In fact, vitamin D has been shown to prevent the growth of melanomas in experimental animals and cultured tissue lines.

An unexpected bonus of vitamin D is that it may also be one of our most important allies in the war against prostate, breast, and colon cancers. Evidence from population studies confirms that people with the greatest lifetime sun exposures have the lowest rates of these cancers.

Skin cancer is a complex disease, with several factors influencing its ultimate course. In laboratory animals, scientists have found that excessive omega 6 fats promote the development of skin cancer—but omega 3 fats slow it down. Furthermore, antioxidants like beta-carotene, vitamin C, and vitamin E tend to prevent the sun's ultraviolet damage to the skin. You can get these same dietary advantages when you adopt the dietary principles I have laid out in the Paleo Diet. (Note: As with many of the diseases we have discussed, proper diet reduces your risk of developing some types of skin cancer, but it cannot completely prevent it.)

Exposure to sunlight is natural for human beings. It is part of our evolutionary heritage. Without sunlight, it is virtually impossible to achieve an adequate intake of vitamin D from the natural foods that were available to our hunter-gatherer ancestors. Our food supply has been a significant source of vitamin D for a very short time—less than a century, when dairy producers began adding it to milk and, later, margarine. Sunlight exposure is healthy as long as it occurs in a slow, gradual, and limited dose over the course of a lifetime.

As you have seen, the Paleo Diet will not only help you get thin; it will also help prevent and treat a broad range of diseases. The Paleo Diet is good medicine!

PART THREE

The Paleo Diet Program

7

Eating Great:
What to Eat,
What to Avoid

Now that I've talked about why the Paleo Diet is the diet nature intended, let's get down to specifics: how do you get started?

This is the best part—it's so easy. You don't have to balance food blocks, weigh portions, keep a food log, or count calories. As I've shown, the basic guidelines of the Paleo Diet are very simple: all the lean meats, poultry, fish, seafood, fruits (except dried fruits), and vegetables (except starchy tubers—primarily, potatoes) you can eat. Because the mainstay of the Paleo Diet is high-quality, low-fat protein, you won't need to feel guilty about eating lean meat, fish, or seafood at every meal. This is exactly what you *should* be doing, along with as many low-glycemic fruits and veggies as you want.

You're about to embark on a diet of enormous and bountiful diversity, fully backed by thousands of clinical nutrition trials and—most important—by 2.5 million years of evolutionary experience. What do you get in return? If you follow the simple nutritional guidelines laid out in this chapter and spelled out in the next two chapters with tempting meal plans and delicious, easy recipes, you will lose weight; reduce your risk of heart disease, cancer, diabetes, and other chronic diseases; and feel energized all day long. And unlike with almost every other diet you can think of, *you won't feel hungry all the time.* You will feel good on this diet, *because this is the only diet that is consistent with your genetic makeup.*

By imitating the diets of our Paleolithic ancestors with foods you can buy at the supermarket or grow in your own garden, you'll be able to reap the health benefits that are your genetic heritage—freedom from obesity, a high energy level, and excellent health.

It is not possible for us to duplicate precisely all the foods that our ancient ancestors ate. Many of these foods no longer exist—such as the mammoth—or they're unavailable commercially, or they just aren't palatable, given our modern tastes and cultural traditions. However, most of the advantages and benefits of the Paleo Diet can easily be obtained from common foods following the general nutritional guidelines observed by our Paleolithic ancestors.

Making the Diet Work for You

It isn't easy to change the habits of a lifetime, and you don't have to do it overnight. You can ease the transition by adopting the three levels of the Paleo Diet. The levels are based on the concept that what you do occasionally won't harm the overall good of what you do most of the time. Does this mean you can cheat? Yes—sometimes. Occasional cheating and digressions may be just what you need to help you stick to the diet the rest of the time, and they won't sidetrack the weight loss and health effects of this diet.

Getting Enough of the Right Foods

As I discussed earlier, there was no single Paleo diet. Our ancient ancestors made the most of their environment wherever they happened to be. For example, the Inuit people were able to live healthy lives, free of chronic diseases, on a diet that derived at least 97 percent of its energy from animal foods. At the other end of the spectrum were groups like the !Kung in Africa, who obtained 65 percent of their daily calories from plant foods (chiefly the mongongo nut). However, most Paleolithic groups fell somewhere in between, with animal foods generally making up around 55–60 percent of the daily caloric intake. On the Paleo Diet, you should attempt to get a little more than half of your calories from lean meat, organ meats, fish, shellfish, and poultry and the rest from plant foods.

Let's take a look at the wonderful, diverse foods that you can eat in unlimited quantities.

Meats

The key word here is "lean." Of course, this includes chicken and fish. But many people are surprised to find that red meat—beef and pork—organ meats, and game meats are also on the list. How can this be? Because, as I discussed earlier, *the Paleo Diet is not a fat-free diet, it's a bad fat–free diet.* As long as the meat is lean, you can eat your fill. Another noteworthy aspect of the meats available on this diet is their great variety. This is a common response as people begin this diet: "I was in a rut before—hamburgers, hot dogs, and pizza. Now I'm planning my meals around all kinds of meats—some I had never tried before, some I'd never even heard of."

In order to get enough protein and calories, you should eat animal food at almost every meal. You can't just eat animal food, however. You must eat fruits and vegetables, too. Here's why: if protein-dense, extremely lean meats and seafood are your main sources of calories, you will get sick—with nausea, diarrhea, and weakness—because your body can't handle this much undiluted protein without something else, either fat or carbohydrates. As we discussed earlier, early Arctic explorers, trappers, and frontiersmen who had no choice but to eat the fat-depleted meat of game animals in the dregs of winter rapidly developed these same symptoms, frequently referred to as "rabbit starvation" or protein toxicity.

The problem, as shown in Dr. Daniel Rudman's laboratory at Emory University in Atlanta, is that the liver can't effectively eliminate the nitrogen caused by the protein overload. For most people, the dietary protein ceiling is 200 to 300 grams a day, or about 30 to 40 percent of the normal daily caloric intake.

On the other hand, eating too many fatty meats can wipe out any health benefits that eating high levels of protein will help you achieve. Paleolithic people couldn't eat fatty meats if they tried—they had nothing like the tubby grain-fed animals that produce our steaks today. Wild game meat contains about 15 to 20 percent of its calories as fat. A lean cut of beef trimmed of all visible fat contains more than double this amount (35 to 40 percent fat). And certain fatty cuts of meats may contain 65 to 80 percent fat.

FAT AND PROTEIN CONTENT
(PERCENTAGE OF TOTAL CALORIES OF MEAT AND FISH)

Meats/Seafood You Can Eat	% Protein	% Fat	Meats to Avoid	% Protein	% Fat
Skinless turkey breasts	94	5	Fat pork chops	49	51
Boiled shrimp	90	10	Lean lamb chops	49	51
Orange roughy	90	10	Pork shoulder roast	45	55
Pollock	90	10	Ham lunch meat	39	54
Broiled lobster	89	5	T-bone steak	36	64
Red snapper	87	13	Chicken thigh/leg	36	63
Dungeness crab	86	10	Ground beef (15% fat)	35	63
Alaskan king crab legs	85	15	Eggs	34	62
Buffalo roast	84	16	Lamb shoulder roast	32	68
Broiled mackerel	82	18	Pork ribs	27	73
Roast venison	81	19	Beef ribs	26	74
Broiled halibut	80	20	Fat lamb chops	25	75
Beef sweetbreads	77	23	Dry salami	23	75
Steamed clams	73	12	Link pork sausage	22	77
Pork tenderloin (lean)	72	28	Bacon	21	78
Beef heart	69	30	Liverwurst	18	79
Broiled tuna	68	32	Bologna	15	81
Veal steak	68	32	Hot dog	14	83
Sirloin beef steak	65	35			
Chicken livers	65	32			
Skinless chicken breasts	63	37			
Beef liver	63	28			
Lean beef flank steak	62	38			
Broiled salmon	62	38			
Lean pork chops	62	38			
Mussels	58	24			

Not only is the total amount of fat higher in commonly consumed fatty meats—such as hamburger, T-bone steak, hot dogs, and lamb chops—than that found in fish and game meat, but the *types* of fat are also quite different. Because most commercially available beef has been feedlot-fattened (mainly with corn and sorghum), it contains low levels of omega 3 fats and high levels of omega 6 fats. This is the wrong mix. When eaten in excess, omega

6 fats are harmful, while omega 3 fats are greatly beneficial. The average Western diet is burdened by high levels of omega 6 fats—which can promote the development of heart disease in many ways. The meats, fish, and seafood you'll be eating on the Paleo Diet are low in fat and high in protein, and they contain the correct balance of omega 3 and omega 6 fats.

What about eggs? Eggs are a relatively high-fat food (62 percent fat, 34 percent protein). Eating too many eggs can promote weight gain and increase blood cholesterol levels. There is no doubt that Paleolithic people would have eaten wild bird eggs whenever they found them. But this wasn't that often. Wild eggs always would have been a seasonal food and would not have been eaten every day. Also, wild bird eggs are nutritionally different from domesticated chicken eggs; they have higher levels of beneficial omega 3 fat and lower levels of certain saturated fats. You should also buy eggs enriched with omega 3 fats.

The high protein of the Paleo Diet is the key to many of its weight-loss benefits. Protein helps you lose weight faster by boosting your metabolism while simultaneously blunting your hunger. And while this is happening, low-fat protein is improving your blood lipid and cholesterol levels, as studies from Dr. Bernard Wolfe's laboratory at the University of Western Ontario have confirmed. Low-fat protein also prevents blood sugar swings and reduces the risk of hypertension, stroke, heart disease, and certain cancers.

Salmon for breakfast? Breakfast is one part of the Paleo Diet that may seem a bit strange at first. In Western countries, breakfast is usually a high-carbohydrate affair, featuring a cereal product (bagel, sweet roll, buttered bread, packaged cereal with milk, oatmeal), coffee or fruit juice, and a piece of fruit. The other common option is the high-fat, "stick to your ribs" breakfast—bacon, sausage, ham, eggs, omelets, hash-brown potatoes, and occasionally steak or pork chops.

Salmon steak and chicken breast aren't on very many breakfast menus. And yet studies indicate that for Paleolithic people, the morning meal was high in protein, was low in carbohydrates and fat, and probably contained "leftovers" from the animal that was killed the day before. A common breakfast on the Paleo Diet, then, might be a cold salmon steak or cold crab (left over from last night's supper) and half a cantaloupe. So go ahead—try fish or meat first thing in the morning. You'll soon find yourself looking trimmer and feeling fitter right at the start of the day.

What to Eat?

Here are the specifics of the Paleo Diet. We'll start with domestic meats. Eat as much as you want for breakfast, lunch, and dinner. Cook the meats simply, without too much added fat—broiling, baking, roasting, sautéing, or browning, then pouring off excess liquid fat, or stir-frying over high heat with a little olive oil (but never deep-fat frying).

Lean Meats

Lean beef (trimmed of visible fat)
- Flank steak
- Top sirloin steak
- Extra-lean hamburger (no more than 7 percent fat, extra fat drained off)
- London broil
- Chuck steak
- Lean veal
- Any other lean cut

Lean pork (trimmed of visible fat)
- Pork loin
- Pork chops
- Any other lean cut

Lean poultry (white meat, skin removed)
- Chicken breast
- Turkey breast
- Game hen breast

Eggs (limit to six to twelve a week)
- Chicken (go for the enriched omega 3 variety)
- Duck
- Goose

Other meats
- Rabbit meat (any cut)
- Goat meat (any cut)

Organ meats
- Beef, lamb, pork, and chicken livers
- Beef, pork, and lamb tongues
- Beef, lamb, and pork marrow
- Beef, lamb, and pork "sweetbreads"

Next, more exotic fare. You may hunt your own or buy locally or via mail order. For a list of exotic-meat suppliers, see chapter 8.

Game meat

- Alligator
- Bear
- Bison (buffalo)
- Caribou
- Elk
- Emu
- Goose
- Kangaroo
- Muscovy duck
- New Zealand cervena deer
- Ostrich
- Pheasant
- Quail
- Rattlesnake
- Reindeer
- Squab
- Turtle
- Venison
- Wild boar
- Wild turkey

Fish

- Bass
- Bluefish
- Cod
- Drum
- Eel
- Flatfish
- Grouper
- Haddock
- Halibut
- Herring
- Mackerel
- Monkfish
- Mullet
- Northern pike
- Orange roughy
- Perch
- Red snapper
- Rockfish
- Salmon
- Scrod
- Shark
- Striped bass
- Sunfish
- Tilapia
- Trout
- Tuna
- Turbot
- Walleye
- Any other commercially available fish

Shellfish

- Abalone
- Clams
- Crab
- Crayfish
- Lobster
- Mussels
- Oysters
- Scallops
- Shrimp

Fruits and Vegetables

It's not easy to get 50 percent of your daily calories from fruits and vegetables because of the high bulk and low caloric density of fruits and salad vegetables. On an average 2,200-calorie diet, you'd have to eat more than 5 pounds of fruits and vegetables a day. Most people are simply unwilling or physiologically unable to consume this much plant food; there is a limit to how much fiber the human gut can hold. However, some plant foods, such as avocados, nuts, seeds, and olive oil, are rich in healthful fats. Eating these in moderate amounts will help you get the calories you need for a balanced diet.

Unless you are severely overweight or obese, you should not worry about how many fresh fruits you eat on the Paleo Diet. Only people with signs and symptoms of metabolic syndrome need to limit consumption of fresh fruits. High-sugar fruits like grapes, bananas, cherries, and mangos should be limited for obese patients or those with signs and symptoms of metabolic syndrome. Low-sugar fruits like berries and melons represent no problems. Check out my Web site: www.the paleodiet.com/nutritional_tools/ fruits_table.html to see a list of fruits that are low in sugars.

Nuts are rich in calories. If you are trying to lose weight, you should eat only about 4 ounces of them a day. Also, except for walnuts, almost all nuts have high levels of omega 6 fats, and if eaten excessively, they can unbalance the ratio of omega 6 to omega 3 fats in your diet.

For ideal health, then, you should eat fruits and vegetables with every meal, along with moderate amounts of nuts, avocados, seeds, and healthful oils (flaxseed and olive). However, just because it's a vegetable doesn't mean it's good—or that it's on the list below. High-carbohydrate, starchy tubers like potatoes are restricted on the Paleo Diet. Also, dried fruit should be eaten only in small amounts because it, too, can produce a high glycemic load (causing a rapid increase in the blood glucose level), particularly when you eat too much of it. When you're hungry or in doubt, start with a high-protein, low-fat food. Remember, lean protein is the most effective nutrient in reducing your appetite and boosting your metabolism to help you burn stored fat.

Fruits

- Apple
- Apricot
- Avocado
- Banana
- Blackberries
- Blueberries
- Boysenberries
- Cantaloupe
- Carambola
- Cassava melon
- Cherimoya
- Cherries

- Cranberries
- Figs
- Gooseberries
- Grapefruit
- Guava
- Grapes
- Honeydew melon
- Kiwi
- Lemon
- Lime
- Lychee
- Mango
- Nectarine
- Orange
- Papaya
- Passion fruit
- Peaches
- Pears
- Persimmon
- Pineapple
- Plums
- Pomegranate
- Raspberries
- Rhubarb
- Star fruit
- Strawberries
- Tangerine
- Watermelon
- All other fruits

Vegetables*

- Artichoke
- Asparagus
- Beet greens
- Beets
- Bell peppers
- Broccoli
- Brussels sprouts
- Cabbage
- Carrots
- Cauliflower
- Celery
- Collards
- Cucumber
- Dandelion
- Eggplant
- Endive
- Green onions
- Kale
- Kohlrabi
- Lettuce
- Mushrooms
- Mustard greens
- Onions
- Parsley
- Parsnip
- Peppers (all kinds)
- Pumpkin
- Purslane
- Radish
- Rutabaga
- Seaweed
- Spinach
- Squash (all kinds)
- Swiss chard
- Tomatillos
- Tomato (actually a fruit, but most people think of it as a vegetable)
- Turnip greens
- Turnips
- Watercress

---

* All, except for starchy tubers like potatoes. Remember, peas and green beans are legumes, and these foods were rarely on Paleo menus.

Nuts and Seeds

Nuts are rich sources of monounsaturated fats. Monounsaturated fats tend to lower cholesterol and reduce the risk of heart disease and may also reduce the risk of certain cancers, including breast cancer. However, because nuts and seeds are such concentrated sources of fat, they have the potential to slow down weight loss, particularly if you're overweight. Again, if you are actively losing weight, you should eat no more than 4 ounces of nuts and seeds a day. Once your metabolism has increased and you've reached your desired weight, you can eat more nuts, particularly walnuts, which have a favorable omega 6 to omega 3 ratio. Note: *Peanuts are legumes, not nuts, and are not on the list.*

- Almonds
- Brazil nuts
- Cashews
- Chestnuts
- Hazelnuts (filberts)
- Macadamia nuts
- Pecans
- Pine nuts
- Pistachios (unsalted)
- Pumpkin seeds
- Sesame seeds
- Sunflower seeds
- Walnuts

Foods You Can Eat in Moderation

Some people are surprised to find alcohol in this next category. There is no evidence to suggest that our Paleolithic ancestors drank any form of alcoholic beverage. And it's abundantly clear, in our own day, that abuse of alcohol—in addition to causing a host of serious behavioral and social problems—can impair your health, damage your liver, and increase your risk of developing many cancers. However, if you currently drink in moderation—if you enjoy an occasional beer or glass of wine—there's no need to give up this pleasure on the Paleo Diet. In fact, numerous scientific studies suggest that moderate alcohol consumption significantly reduces the risk of dying from heart disease and other illnesses. Wine in particular, when consumed in moderation, has been shown to have many beneficial health effects. A glass of wine before or during dinner may help improve your insulin sensitivity and reduce your appetite. Wine is also an appetizing, salt-free ingredient that adds flavor to many meat and vegetable dishes. Note: If you have an autoimmune disease, you should avoid alcoholic beverages and other yeast-containing foods. (For more information, see chapter 6.)

Oils
- Olive, avocado, walnut, and flaxseed oils (use in moderation—4 tablespoons or less a day when weight loss is of primary importance)

Beverages
- Diet sodas (These often contain artificial sweeteners such as aspartame and saccharine, which may be harmful; you're better off drinking bottled and mineral waters.)
- Coffee
- Tea
- Wine (two 4-ounce glasses. Note: Don't buy "cooking wine," which is loaded with salt.)
- Beer (one 12-ounce serving)
- Spirits (4 ounces)

Paleo Sweets
- Dried fruits (no more than 2 ounces a day, particularly if you are trying to lose weight)
- Nuts mixed with dried and fresh fruits (no more than 4 ounces of nuts and 2 ounces of dried fruit a day, particularly if you are trying to lose weight)

Foods You Should Avoid

I've spent a lot of time talking about why the foods in this next category should not be part of your diet. (You don't have to stop cold turkey, though; you can gradually wean them from your diet, as I'll discuss below.) Except for honey, refined sugars were nonexistent in Paleo diets; so were dairy products and excess salt. Almost all processed food is a mix of three or four of the following: sugar, some form of starch (wheat, potatoes, corn, rice), fat or oil, dairy products, salt, and flavorings. Because most processed foods are made with refined grains, starches, and sugars, they are high-glycemic items and can cause large swings in blood sugar levels. Most modern cereal- and sugar-based processed foods adversely affect insulin metabolism and are associated with a greater risk of obesity, heart disease, diabetes, high blood pressure, and other chronic health problems.

Just because these foods are not part of the diet, you don't have to banish them from your life forever. But you should try to avoid them most of the time.

Dairy Foods

- All processed foods made with any dairy products
- Butter
- Cheese
- Cream
- Dairy spreads
- Frozen yogurt
- Ice cream
- Ice milk
- Low-fat milk
- Nonfat dairy creamer
- Powdered milk
- Skim milk
- Whole milk
- Yogurt

Cereal Grains

- Barley (barley soup, barley bread, and all processed foods made with barley)
- Corn (corn on the cob, corn tortillas, corn chips, cornstarch, corn syrup)
- Millet
- Oats (steel-cut oats, rolled oats, and all processed foods made with oats)
- Rice (brown rice, white rice, ramen, rice noodles, basmati rice, rice cakes, rice flour, and all processed foods made with rice)
- Rye (rye bread, rye crackers, and all processed foods made with rye)
- Sorghum
- Wheat (bread, rolls, muffins, noodles, crackers, cookies, cake, doughnuts, pancakes, waffles, pasta, spaghetti, lasagna, wheat tortillas, pizza, pita bread, flat bread, and all processed foods made with wheat or wheat flour)
- Wild rice

Cereal-Grainlike Seeds

- Amaranth
- Buckwheat
- Quinoa

Legumes

- All beans (adzuki beans, black beans, broad beans, fava beans, field beans, garbanzo beans, horse beans, kidney beans, lima beans, mung beans, navy beans, pinto beans, red beans, string beans, white beans)
- Black-eyed peas
- Chickpeas
- Lentils
- Peas
- Peanut butter
- Peanuts
- Snow peas
- Sugar snap peas
- Soybeans and all soybean products, including tofu

Starchy Vegetables

- Starchy tubers
- Cassava root
- Manioc
- Potatoes and all potato products (French fries, potato chips, etc.)
- Sweet potatoes
- Tapioca pudding
- Yams

Salt-Containing Foods

- Almost all commercial salad dressings and condiments
- Bacon
- Cheese
- Deli meats
- Frankfurters
- Ham
- Hot dogs
- Ketchup
- Olives
- Pickled foods
- Pork rinds
- Processed meats
- Salami
- Salted nuts
- Salted spices
- Sausages
- Smoked, dried, and salted fish and meat
- Virtually all canned meats and fish (unless they are unsalted or unless you soak and drain them)

Fatty Meats

- Bacon
- Bacon bits
- Bologna
- Breakfast sausage
- Chicken and turkey skin
- Chicken wings
- Deli meats
- Fatty lamb chops
- Fatty pork chops
- Pepperoni
- Pork sausage
- Salami
- Spam

Soft Drinks and Fruit Juices

- All sugary soft drinks
- Canned, bottled, and freshly squeezed fruit drinks (which lack the fiber of fresh fruit and have a much higher glycemic index)

Sweets

- Candy
- Honey
- Sugars

As you can see, there's a bounty of wonderful foods you can eat on the Paleo Diet, so you'll never get bored. Use your imagination and have fun with these delicious foods.

8

The Paleo Diet
User's Manual

Stocking Your Refrigerator and Pantry

You know those diets where you have to buy *their food*, in *their packaging*, at *their stores*? This is different. You don't need to buy any special foods to follow the Paleo Diet. Just about everything you need is right in your local supermarket—particularly if it has a health food section. Even if you live in a rural area, the basics of the diet—lean meats, fish, fresh fruits, and vegetables—can be found in small grocery stores. If you choose, you can order specialty oils and game meats through the mail (some suppliers are listed below). But you don't need anything out of the ordinary to get started.

Look for Lean Meats

The mainstay of the Paleo Diet is lean animal foods. Always choose the leanest cut of meat you can find.

Beef

If you can get it—it might be at the butcher's counter, not out in the main meat aisle—"range-fed" is better than grain-fed beef because it's leaner, and it has a better ratio of omega 6 to omega 3 fatty acids. Note: The words "natural beef" are no guarantee that the animal hasn't been fattened with grains (or pumped full of antibiotics, for that matter); check with your butcher. A simple visual inspection of the fat on any cut of meat lets you know if the animal was raised on pasture or on grains. Pasture-produced meat has fat that is orange to dark yellow in color, whereas grain-produced meat has fat that appears white.

Poultry

"Free-range" chickens are almost always better than broiler chickens, because—like range-fed beef—they're not as fat. Here, too, the natural foraging diet (of insects, worms, and wild plants) guarantees a healthful ratio of omega 6 to omega 3 fatty acids. Free-range chickens can be found in many upscale or health-oriented supermarkets.

Turkey

Turkey breast is one of the best and cheapest sources of very lean meat—it's even leaner than most game meat—and fortunately, it's available almost everywhere. *Tip: Before you cook very lean domestic meats, rub them with olive oil. This will add flavor and help keep them moist during cooking.*

Pork

Some pork is *even leaner than chicken.* Lean pork tenderloin, for instance, has 28 percent fat compared to skinless chicken breasts at 37 percent. Naturally grown pork—similar to free-range chickens—is leaner, too.

Other Choices

What about organ meats? Many people mistakenly think organ meats are fatty. Organ meats are low in fat and are rich sources of vitamins, minerals, and omega 3 fat. Bone marrow is another overlooked food that's seldom eaten in the United States but is considered a delicacy in Europe. Even though it contains about 80 percent fat by weight, almost 75 percent of the fat is monounsaturated—which means that marrow is a good fat that won't raise your cholesterol.

As for lamb, if you can find grass-fed, free-range meat, go for it. The type of lamb produced in Australia and New Zealand is leaner than American grain-fed lamb and contains more healthful omega 3 fats. Remember, leaner, grass-produced meat is the key to making this lifelong nutrition plan work for you.

One of the best online resources for locating healthy, naturally produced, grass-fed meats is my friend and colleague Jo Robinson's Eatwild Web site: www.eatwild.com. Jo's Web site is an incredible cornucopia of information that will help you locate a reliable producer of grass-fed, natural meat in your local region. Eatwild's Directory of Farms lists more than 1,300 pasture-based farms, with more farms being added regularly. It is the most comprehensive source for grass-fed meat in the United States and Canada. For your convenience, Jo provides customers with contact information of suppliers who will ship their products to you.

Wild Game Meat—at a Gourmet Store Near You

In the United States, it's illegal to harvest wild game meat for commercial use. This means that the game meat you can buy from specialty suppliers (some are listed below) didn't come from the wild, but from a ranch or a farm—where these animals graze freely in large fenced or open areas. Most game animals are raised in free-range conditions. Like its wild counterpart, this game meat is quite low in fat and maintains a healthful balance of omega 6 and omega 3 fatty acids.

You can find buffalo and sometimes rabbit meat in many supermarkets—especially the upscale or health-oriented ones—and more exotic fare in specialty meat and butcher shops. Your local butcher may be able to order game meat as well, but be prepared—it isn't cheap. If you are a hunter (or if you know someone who is, who would be willing to help out), you can save a lot of money by acquiring wild meat yourself.

Like all very lean meat, game meat is a bit tricky to cook. It's also easy to ruin so that it loses its texture and appeal.

It also helps to rub the meat thoroughly with olive oil before cooking and keep basting it as it cooks. If you grill game meat, keep it on the rare side, baste it often with olive oil or marinades, and it will be tender.

The secret to making game tender—and not rubbery or leathery—is to cook it very slowly over low heat in a covered dish with a bit of water

If you've never tasted game meat, you may be in for a big surprise. Some game meats, like buffalo and elk, taste a lot like lean beef, but with a sweeter, richer flavor. Others, like antelope or sage hen, can have a distinctively pungent flavor—the telltale "gamey" taste. This gamey flavor is actually a good sign; it results from the increased levels of omega 3 fats in the meat, plus various wild plants in the animal's diet. It also indicates that the game meat you're eating is healthy, with a good balance of omega 6 and omega 3 fats. If you're not used to game meat's distinctive flavors—or if you never want to get used to it—overnight marinating can do wonders.

Here are some mail-order suppliers that specialize in the sale of game meat:

Game Sales International
P.O. Box 7719
Loveland, CO 80537
Phone: (800) 729-2090
Fax: (970) 669-9041
www.gamesalesintl.com

Exotic Meat Market
130 Walnut Avenue, Unit A-18
Perris, CA 92571
Phone: (951) 345-4623
http://exoticmeatmarket.com

Hills Foods Ltd.
Unit 130 Glacier Street
Coquitlam, British Columbia
Canada V3K 5Z6
Phone: (604) 472-1500
www.hillsfoods.com

Grande Natural Meat
P.O. Box 10
Del Norte, Colorado 81132

Phone: (888) 338-4581
www.elkusa.com

Mount Royal Game Meat
3902 N. Main
Houston, TX 77009
Phone: (800) 730-3337
www.mountroyal.com

Polarica (West Coast)
105 Quint Street
San Francisco, CA 94124
Phone: (800) 426-3872
www.polarica.com

Broken Arrow Ranch
3296 Junction Highway
Ingram, TX 78025
Phone: (800) 962-4263
www.brokenarrowranch.com

Exotic Meats USA
1330 Capita Blvd.
Reno, NV 89502
Phone: (800) 444-5687
www.exoticmeatsandmore.com

Southern Game Meat (Kangaroo)
Unit 1/5 Stanton Road
Seven Hills
NSW 2147 Australia
Phone: 61-2-8825-8350
www.sgm.com.au

Fish and Seafood

Nutritionally speaking, fish and seafood are a lot like humanity's original staple food—lean game meat. They're high in protein, low in total fat, and typically high in omega 3 fats. Many scientific studies have shown that regular fish consumption reduces bad LDL cholesterol and triglycerides while simultaneously increasing the good HDL cholesterol. The omega 3 fats in fish also prevent the heart from going into irregular, uncontrolled beating patterns called "arrhythmias," which can be fatal. *Fish is just plain good for you.* It lowers your risk of heart attack, stroke, and type 2 diabetes. By eating fish and seafood regularly, you can significantly reduce your risk of dying from the number one killer of all Americans—heart disease.

Unfortunately, there's a downside, and it has nothing to do with fish and seafood, but with our own environment. Fish and seafood are often contaminated with heavy metals, particularly mercury; by polychlorinated biphenyls (PCBs); and by pesticides such as DDT and dieldrin. The places where fish live—oceans, rivers, lakes, and streams—are also the dumping grounds for many of these potentially harmful chemicals. Once in the water, these toxins seep into the sediments and then into the plants. They're ingested by the tiny animals that form the base of the food chain. Little fish eat plants and tiny animals, and bigger fish eat little fish. Heavy metals and fat-soluble pesticides can become concentrated in older fish, in predatory fish, and in fatty species of fish.

Mercury finds its way into our waterways as a by-product of fuel-burning and through household and industrial wastes. Bacteria in the water convert mercury into the toxic compound methylmercury. When we eat mercury-contaminated fish, we can develop mercury poisoning, which can damage the brain and the nervous system. The good news is that most of the time, the amount of mercury we get from fish is quite small. And the amount of mercury that you can potentially accumulate by eating fish three or four times a week is tiny compared to how much you could get by industrial or occupational exposure.

For healthy people, regular fish consumption poses virtually no risk to brain or nervous system function. It's safe even for pregnant women and very young children, concludes a comprehensive study conducted by Dr. Philip Davidson and colleagues at the University of Rochester School of Medicine and Dentistry in New York. Their findings, published in the *Journal of the American Medical Association,* come from a nine-year study conducted in the Republic of the Seychelles, an island nation in the Indian Ocean, where most people eat fish nearly a dozen times a week and have mercury levels *about ten times higher* than those of most Americans. In fact, no harmful effects were seen in the nervous systems and behavior of children at mercury levels *up to twenty times* the average American level.

It is a worrisome fact that we live in a polluted world, and most of us are exposed to a host of toxic compounds. However, the greatest risk to your health is not from environmental pollutants, but from heart disease, diabetes, obesity, stroke, and the associated health disorders of metabolic syndrome. *Eating fish protects you not only from these diseases but from all causes of death, including cancer.* Because fish is one of our greatest sources of omega 3 fats, it can also help prevent depression and improve your mood, as my friend and colleague Dr. Joseph Hibbeln of the National Institutes of Health has shown. In short, fish should be part of your diet.

You should still be prudent when you shop for fish and seafood. Here are a few ways you can minimize your risk of eating contaminated fish:

- Avoid freshwater fish taken from lakes and rivers—particularly the Great Lakes and other polluted, industrialized areas.
- Choose fish that come from cleaner waters, such as the Pacific Ocean and in Alaska.
- Eat mainly smaller, nonpredatory species such as flounder, herring, sardines, sole, pollock, catfish, halibut, and clams.
- Eat big fish—swordfish, shark, and tuna—sparingly. These long-lived predatory fish tend to accumulate more mercury.

Fortunately, over the long run, the Paleo Diet's many fruits and vegetables—and their disease-fighting antioxidants—can help prevent cancers and health problems that are a direct result of our environmentally polluted world.

How to Be a Savvy Shopper for Fish

Yet the possibility of environmental contamination isn't the only thing you have to worry about when you eat fresh fish and seafood. Another, much bigger concern is simply whether the fish has gone bad. Improper handling and warm temperatures offer great potential for bacterial contamination and spoilage as fish makes its way from wherever it was caught to its eventual place of sale. The freshness clock begins to tick immediately: most fish have a shelf life of seven to twelve days once they're out of the water. But fish often remain on a boat for five to six days after they're caught. They may spend another day or two in transit from the processor/wholesaler to the marketplace—and then may sit on a retailer's display counter for several days more before they are sold. If the fish get too warm during any stage of transport, they'll spoil even faster. Bacteria are the main culprits in the spoilage process, but enzymes in the fish tissue and even atmospheric oxygen can contribute. Fortunately, spoiled fish release a pungent warning—a compound called "trimethylamine," which causes the telltale fishy odor associated with bad fish.

Fresh fish is practically odorless. If a fish smells, spoilage is most likely well under way—so stay away from smelly fish. Here are some other tips:

- If you're buying whole fish—and it passes the odor test—check the gills. If they're bright red and moist, the fish is probably fine. If the gills are brown or clumped together, the fish has been on the shelf too long.
- Buy fish last. If you're making a prolonged excursion to the grocery store, don't get the fish first and then let it sit in the cart for an hour while you get everything else on the list. Select it, pay for it, go home—and immediately refrigerate the fish *in its original package in the coldest part of your refrigerator.* Try to eat the fish no more than a day after you buy it.
- To protect yourself from bacterial contamination, wash the fish in cold water and then cook it thoroughly, until it's opaque and flakes easily with a fork. This is important: bacteria and parasites sometimes live in raw fish. But if you cook the fish completely, you'll minimize your chances of getting sick—even if you inadvertently eat fish that has partially spoiled.
- Avoid eating raw fish of any kind for the reasons above.
- If you can't eat fresh fish within a day or two of buying it, freeze it. Freezing completely stops bacterial growth. However, once the fish thaws, the same deterioration process starts again.
- Be careful when you buy fish labeled "previously frozen." This may be once-fresh fish that wasn't bought, went past its expiration date, was frozen by the retailer, and was thawed again for quick sale.
- Look for light-colored, cottony spots on the fish—they're freezer burns. Sometimes frozen fish is allowed to thaw and then is refrozen, sometimes several times. Also look for ice crystal coatings—and walk away if you find them. These are

fish you don't want to buy. The highest-quality frozen fish are caught at sea and then quick-frozen individually on board the ship. (Often, there's a label to this effect, saying that the fish was "frozen at sea.")

What about Farm-Raised Fish?

It's called "aquaculture." Many species of fish and shellfish—including salmon, trout, catfish, tilapia, carp, eels, shrimp, and crayfish—are produced in closed waters and ponds and fed soy- and cereal-based chows. This is similar to the situation of feedlot-fed cattle. What they eat causes their own meat to be low or deficient in the beneficial omega 3 fatty acids that help make fish so good for us. Numerous scientific studies have demonstrated the omega 3 fatty acid inferiority of farmed fish compared to wild fish.

Farmed fish are usually cheaper to bring to market than wild fish. In the United States, trout—unless you have caught it yourself in the wild—is almost always farmed. Fresh, wild salmon has a marvelous flavor; most farmed salmon is bland-tasting. Decide for yourself. Note: Some farmed fish is labeled as such; most is not. If you don't know, ask your grocer.

Should You Eat Canned Fish?

Canned tuna is America's favorite fish by far. But the canning process causes a number of problems, the least of which is a loss of fresh flavor. This is what happens: the tuna is cooked at high temperatures and then sealed in a can containing salt, vegetable oil, water, or a combination of these three ingredients. The canning process removes 99 percent of the vitamin A found in fresh tuna, 97 percent of the vitamin B_1, 86 percent of the vitamin B_2, 45 percent of the niacin, and 59 percent of the vitamin B_6. It also increases the level of oxidized cholesterol in the fish, specifically a molecule called "25-hydroxycholesterol" that is extremely destructive to the linings of arterial blood vessels—so destructive that oxidized cholesterol is routinely fed to laboratory animals to accelerate artery clogging in order to test theories of heart disease. In animal models of atherosclerosis and heart disease, only 0.3 percent of the dietary cholesterol needs to be in the form of oxidized cholesterol to cause premature damage to the arterial linings.

To complete the degradation of this formerly healthy food, the tuna is packed with salt water or vegetable oils, which usually are high in omega 6 fatty acids. If you have the choice, always choose fresh or frozen fish over canned fish. If you do eat canned tuna, try to find brands that are packed in water only (no salt) or in more healthful oils, such as olive. (Most water-packed tuna contains added salt, but this can be removed by soaking the tuna in a shallow pan filled with tap water and then rinsing the fish in a colander under a running tap.)

Eggs: Good or Bad?

Eggs are healthful foods; our Paleolithic ancestors ate them seasonally, because they just weren't available all the time. Several recent studies have shown that eating one egg a day has no discernible effect on your blood cholesterol level and does not increase your risk of heart disease. So go ahead—enjoy a couple of eggs for breakfast every few days.

There's more good news on the egg front: you can buy chicken eggs that, like the wild bird eggs our ancestors ate, have high levels of omega 3 fatty acids. These enriched eggs—produced when chicken are fed omega 3–enriched feeds—are nutritionally superior and are available at many supermarkets and health food stores.

Because eggs are one of our richest dietary sources of cholesterol, the way they're cooked influences the level of oxidized cholesterol—which can damage the cells lining your arteries and increase your risk of developing atherosclerosis and heart disease. High heat—like that of a griddle—produces more oxidized cholesterol than slow cooking: poaching, hard-boiling, or baking. When you have the choice, avoid fried eggs.

A recent study demonstrated that eggs from free-range hens had up to ⅓ less cholesterol, ¼ less saturated fat, ⅔ more vitamin A, 2 times more omega 3 fatty acids, 3 times more vitamin E, and 7 times more beta-carotene, than battery-cage eggs.

Similar to the situation with grass-fed, free-range meats, eggs produced from chickens allowed to live and forage freely are more nutritious and healthful than are their factory-produced counterparts. One of the first poultry farmers to recognize the superiority of free-range eggs was my friend George Bass. You can sample George's eggs at his Web site for the Country Hen below. I also recommend that you visit Jo Robinson's Web site, www.eatwild.com, to find a local producer of free-range eggs near your home.

The Country Hen
P.O. Box 333
Hubbardston, MA 01452
Phone: (978) 928-5333
countryhen.com

How to Make the Most of Fruits and Vegetables

One of the first changes you'll notice when you start the Paleo Diet is the large amounts of fresh fruits and veggies that you will need to keep on hand. Note: To help produce stay fresh longer, keep fruits and vegetables covered in plastic bags in your refrigerator.

The constant need to replenish your fresh produce supply gives you a good excuse to explore new venues. Try going to local farmers' markets in your area. They're wonderful sources of wholesome, fresh, and delicious fruits and vegetables. They may even inspire you to try growing your own vegetables at home. Also, take this opportunity to try out-of-the-ordinary fruits and vegetables (many are included in the recipes and meal plans in this book). You may want to look for exotic produce in Asian, Far Eastern, and ethnic markets if there are any in your community. As you gradually wean yourself from salty, sugary, and starchy foods, your taste buds will become attuned to the subtle flavors and textures of wonderful real foods.

To be on the safe side, be sure to wash all produce before you eat it (even if it comes in a bag that says it's been washed). Like fish, fresh produce can contain trace residues of pesticides, heavy metals, or other pollutants. The Food and Drug Administration has monitored the levels of contaminants in the U.S. food supply for almost forty years in a program called the Total Diet Study (you can read about it on the Web at: vm.cfsan.fda.gov/~comm/tds-toc.html). The study, which began in 1961, periodically examines more than 230 foods from eight regional metropolitan areas to determine which hidden ingredients—and how much of them—we're getting in our food. Since its inception, the study has found that our average daily intake of all toxic contaminants—including pesticides, industrial chemicals, heavy metals, and radioactive materials—is well below acceptable limits. Of course, it would be even better if our average daily intake of contaminants were zero, and we could rest assured that our food was completely free of any pollution—but it's pretty safe to say that this will not happen any time soon.

> If you are concerned about pesticide exposure, artificial fertilizer, and other food safety issues, you may want to seek organically grown produce whenever possible, although it's a bit more expensive

The bottom line is that fruits and vegetables have much to offer—antioxidants, vitamins, minerals, and all the healing benefits we've discussed in this book. We can't do without them; more than that, they need to play a starring role in our diet.

Nuts and Seeds

Nuts and seeds are a good adjunct to the Paleo Diet, but they've got a lot of fat, so you need to eat them in moderation. Too many fatty foods—even beneficial nuts and seeds—can rapidly upset your balance of essential dietary fats and derail your weight-loss progress. Throughout the book, we've talked about the omegas—omega 6 and omega 3. One kind—omega 6 fats—is not good for you when eaten in excess. The other kind—omega 3 fats—can make you healthier in many ways. The ideal ratio of omega 6 to omega 3 fats should be between 2 and 3 to 1. For most Americans, unfortunately, it's between 10 and 15 to 1. All nuts and seeds—except for walnuts and possibly macadamia nuts—have unacceptably high omega 6 to omega 3 ratios. This is why you must eat them in small amounts.

Omega 6 to Omega 3 Fat Ratio in Nuts and Seeds

Nut or Seed	Omega 6 to Omega 3 Ratio
Walnuts	4.2
Macadamia nuts	6.3
Pecans	20.9

Nut or Seed	Omega 6 to Omega 3 Ratio
Pine nuts	31.6
Cashews	47.6
Pistachio nuts	51.9
Hazelnuts (filberts)	90.0
Pumpkin seeds	114.4
Brazil nuts	377.9
Sunflower seeds	472.9
Almonds	extremely high (no detectable omega 3 fats)
Peanuts (not a nut but a legume)	extremely high (no detectable omega 3 fats)

But nuts are part of the Paleo Diet. They're high in mono-unsaturated fats and have been shown in numerous clinical trials to lower cholesterol. This is why they're on the diet *in moderate amounts,* so that you can benefit from the good things nuts have to offer. But the high quantities of omega 6 fats in these nuts can also predispose you to heart disease—because they displace the omega 3 fats, which are known to prevent fatal heartbeat irregularities, decrease blood clotting, lower blood triglyceride levels, and reduce the inflammatory profile of prostaglandins and leukotrienes (hormonelike substances that control the inflammation process). Omega 3 fats have also been shown to lessen the symptoms of many inflammatory and autoimmune diseases, including arthritis and inflammatory bowel disease.

Peanuts are forbidden. As mentioned, they are not nuts at all; they're legumes—and legumes contain lectins and other antinutrients that can adversely affect your health, particularly if you are suffering from an autoimmune disorder.

Important note: Many people are allergic to nuts, and pine nuts can be particularly troublesome for some people. Listen to your body carefully as you begin the Paleo Diet and fine-tune the diet to your specific health needs. Although nuts and seeds are true Paleo foods—and were certainly part of the diets of our ancient ancestors—they were not the staples.

When you shop for nuts:

- Try to buy raw, unsalted nuts. You can find them in their natural state at most supermarkets in the late summer and early fall when they come into season.

- If you don't like cracking nuts, you can find packaged, hulled nuts at some supermarkets and most health food stores. However, read the package label. Hulled nuts are sometimes coated with trans fat–containing oils to increase their shelf life.
- When in doubt, go for walnuts. They have the best omega 6 to omega 3 ratio and are your healthiest choice for a snack food or to use in other dishes. Other nuts should be considered garnishes in salads and other dishes, rather than eaten in quantity.

Purchasing Oils

Vegetable oils were obviously not a component of any pre-agricultural or hunter-gatherer diet, simply because the technology to produce them did not exist. Oils made from walnuts, almonds, olives, sesame seeds, and flaxseeds were first produced using crude presses between 5,000 and 6,000 years ago. However, except for olive oil, most early oil use was for nonfood purposes, such as illumination, lubrication, and medicine. It wasn't until the beginning of the twentieth century, with the advent of mechanically driven steel expellers and hexane extraction processes, that vegetable oils started to contribute significantly to the caloric content of the Western diet. Today vegetable oils used in cooking, salad oils, margarine, shortening, and processed foods supply 17.6 percent of the total daily energy intake in the U.S. diet. The enormous infusion of vegetable oils into the Western diet, starting in the early 1900s, represents the greatest single factor responsible for elevating the dietary omega 6 to omega 3 ratio to its current and unhealthful value of 10 to 1. In hunter-gatherer diets, the omega 6 to omega 3 ratio was closer to 2 to 1. If we use the evolutionary template exclusively, vegetable oils should probably constitute a minimal part of modern-day Paleo diets.

So, if this is the case, why should we not eliminate all vegetable oils from our diet?

I still believe that certain oils can be used to cook with and add flavor when making condiments, dressings, and marinades. Simply stated, there are four oils (flaxseed, walnut, olive, and avocado) that can promote health and facilitate your getting the correct balance of good fats into your diet. Because hunter-gatherers ate the entire carcasses of wild animals (tongue, eyes, brains, marrow, liver, gonads, intestines, kidneys, and so on) and relished fatty plant foods (nuts and seeds), they did not have to worry about the correct balance of fatty acids in their diet. It came out correctly in the wash.

For most of us, the thought of eating organs is not only repulsive, but is also not practical as we simply do not have access to wild game. Consequently, by eating lean meats, fish, and seafood, along with healthful oils, nuts, and seeds, you can get the correct balance of fatty acids in your diet.

As you can see from the table on page 134, only three vegetable oils have omega 6 to omega 3 ratios of less than 3. These are flaxseed (0.24), canola (2.0), and mustard seed (2.6). Although I originally recommended mustard seed oil in the first edition of *The Paleo Diet*, I can no longer make this recommendation because of its high erucic acid (a long-chain monounsaturated fatty acid) concentration of 41.2 percent. Consumption of large quantities of erucic acid in laboratory animals causes adverse changes in their heart structure and function and other organs.

This leaves only two vegetable oils (canola and flaxseed) that do not contribute to an elevated intake of omega 6 fatty acids. A number of epidemiological (population) studies have shown a higher risk of developing prostate cancer with an increased consumption of alpha linolenic acid (ALA), a major fatty acid found in both canola and flaxseed oil. However, epidemiological studies are notorious for their conflicting results. For every six studies that support one nutritional concept, you can often find half a dozen more that conclude precisely the opposite. Such is the case linking ALA and flaxseed oil to an increased prostate cancer risk. A series of the most recent epidemiological studies was unable to statistically show that ALA consumption increased prostate cancer risk. More important, in experiments in which animals were fed flaxseed oil, the flaxseed actually inhibited the growth and development of prostate cancer. The case supporting flaxseed oil as a promoter of prostate cancer is currently based solely on epidemiological evidence and therefore remains inconclusive because of the total lack of confirming experimental evidence. Because the majority of epidemiological studies support the notion that ALA is protective against cardiovascular disease, flaxseed oil should still be viewed as healthful.

Since the original publication of *The Paleo Diet* in 2002, I have reversed my view of canola oil and can no longer support its consumption or use. Let me explain why. Canola oil comes from the seeds of the rape plant (*Brassica rapa* or *Brassica campestris*), which is a close relative of broccoli, cabbage, Brussels sprouts, and kale. Clearly, humans have eaten cabbage and its relatives since prior to historical times, and I still strongly support the consumption of these health-promoting vegetables. The concentrated oil from the seeds of *Brassica* plants is another story.

In its original form, rape plants produced a seed oil that contained high concentrations (20 to 50 percent) of erucic acid (a monounsaturated fatty acid labeled 22:1n9), which I have previously explained is toxic and which causes a wide variety of pathological changes in laboratory animals. In the early 1970s, plant breeders from Canada developed a strain of rape plant that produced a seed with less than 2 percent erucic acid (hence the name canola oil). The erucic acid content of commercially available canola oil averages 0.6 percent. Despite its low erucic acid content, however, a number of experiments in the 1970s showed that even at low concentrations (2.0 percent and 0.88 percent), canola oil fed to rats could still produce minor heart scarring that was considered "pathological."

A series of recent rat studies of low-erucic canola oil conducted by Dr. Ohara and colleagues at the Hatano Research Institute in Japan reported kidney injuries, as well as increases in blood sodium levels and abnormal changes to a hormone, aldosterone, that regulates blood pressure. Other negative effects of canola oil consumption in animals at 10 percent of calories include decreased litter sizes, behavioral changes, and liver injury. A number of recent human studies of canola/rapeseed oil by Dr. Poiikonen and colleagues at the University of Tempere in Finland have shown it to be a potent allergen in adults and children and indicate that it may cause allergic cross-reactions from other environmental allergens in children with atopic dermatitis (skin rashes).

Based on these up-to-date studies in both humans and animals, I prefer to be on the safe side and can no longer recommend canola oil.

Both olive oil and avocado oil are high (73.9 and 70.6 percent, respectively) in cholesterol-lowering monounsaturated fatty acids but have less than favorable omega 6 to omega 3 ratios of 11.7 and 13.5. Consequently, excessive consumption of both of these oils without adequate intake of long-chain omega 3 fatty acids (EPA plus DHA) will derail an otherwise healthy diet. I recommend that you get 1.0 to 2.0 grams of EPA and DHA per day in your diet from either fish or fish oil capsules. Because avocado oil is difficult to find and expensive, that pretty much leaves olive oil as the staple for cooking, salad dressings, and marinades.

If you can afford it, I recommend that you always choose extra-virgin olive oil, because this grade of oil is produced by physical means only, without chemical treatment, and it contains the highest concentrations of polyphenolic compounds, which protect against cancer, heart disease, and inflammation.

Although peanut oil has been promoted as a healthy, cholesterol-lowering oil because of its high monounsaturated fat content (46 percent of total fat), it has turned out to be one of the most atherogenic (artery-clogging) of all oils. In fact, it is routinely used to induce coronary artery atherosclerosis in monkeys and other laboratory animals. It's not clear exactly why this happens. Some scientific evidence suggests that peanut lectins (proteins that bind to carbohydrates) may be responsible for this effect.

Because soybean oil also contains residual lectin activity (SBA) and maintains a marginal (7.5) omega 6 to omega 3 ratio, it can't be recommended as a staple oil, either. A similar argument can be made for wheat germ oil, which has a marginal omega 6 to omega 3 ratio of 7.9 but also contains large quantities of the lectin WGA, one of the most widely studied and potentially most damaging of all the dietary lectins.

Coconut meat, oil, and milk are traditional foods of indigenous people who live in the tropics. These foods have high amounts of a saturated fat called lauric acid, which is known to elevate blood cholesterol concentrations—a risk factor for cardiovascular disease in modern Westernized populations. Paradoxically, traditional cultures that consume coconut foods have a minimal or nonexistent incidence of heart disease, stroke, or cardiovascular complications normally associated with eating high levels of saturated fats, such as the lauric acid found in coconut food products.

Lauric acid apparently exerts a protective effect in our bodies by eliminating gut bacteria that increase intestinal permeability, a risk factor for cardiovascular disease via heightened chronic low-level inflammation. Based on the evidence of traditional Pacific Islanders who consume coconut, it appears that this food does not present a risk for cardiovascular disease when included as a component of modern Paleo Diets. Let your palate go back to the islands and enjoy the delicious health benefits of this traditional plant food.

SALAD AND COOKING OILS

	Omega 6 to Omega 3	% MUFA	% PUFA	% SAT
1. Flaxseed oil	0.24	20.2	66.0	9.4
2. Canola oil	2.00	58.9	29.6	7.1
3. Mustard seed oil	2.60	59.2	21.2	11.6
4. Walnut oil	5.08	22.8	63.3	9.1
5. Olive oil	13.1	72.5	8.4	13.5
6. Avocado oil	13.0	67.9	13.5	11.6
7. Almond oil	no Omega 3	69.9	17.4	8.2
8. Apricot kernel oil	no Omega 3	60.0	29.3	6.3
9. Coconut oil	no Omega 3	5.8	1.8	86.5
10. Corn oil	83	24.2	58.7	12.7
11. Cottonseed oil	258	17.8	51.9	25.9
12. Grapeseed oil	696	16.1	69.9	9.6
13. Hazelnut oil	no Omega 3	78.0	10.2	7.4
14. Oat oil	21.9	35.1	40.9	19.6
15. Palm oil	45.5	37.0	9.3	49.3
16. Peanut oil	no Omega 3	46.2	32.0	16.9
17. Rice bran oil	20.9	39.3	35.0	19.7
18. Safflower oil	no Omega 3	14.4	74.6	6.2
19. Sesame oil	137	39.7	41.7	14.1
20. Soybean oil	7.5	23.3	57.9	14.4
21. Sunflower oil	no Omega 3	19.5	65.7	10.3
22. Tomato seed oil	22.1	22.8	53.1	19.7
23. Wheat germ oil	7.9	15.1	61.7	18.8

MUFA = monounsaturated fat, PUFA = polyunsaturated fat, SAT = saturated fat.

Spices

One of the key elements of the Paleo Diet is to cut way down on your use of salt—or, better yet, cut it out entirely. This doesn't mean you need to eat bland, tasteless food—far from it. If you haven't already plunged into the wonderful world of spices, now's your chance.

Lemon crystals and lemon pepper are good replacements for salt, and they give food a mouthwatering zing. There are also several good salt substitutes, commercially available spice mixes designed to take the place of salt. Note: Check the labels; sometimes spice mixes contain cornstarch, hydrolyzed wheat proteins, or other grain and legume products.

Some people—particularly if they are suffering from an autoimmune disease—should stay away from spices made from chili peppers (cayenne pepper and paprika). This botanical family of spices contains a substance called "capsaicin." Studies by Dr. Erika Jensen-Jarolim and colleagues at University Hospital in Vienna, Austria, have shown that capsaicin increases intestinal permeability and may play a role in the development and progression of certain autoimmune diseases. Again, let your body serve as your guide: if a spice seems to be irritating your system or causing problems, don't use it.

The good news is that most spices are easily digestible and well tolerated and add subtle flavors and overtones to almost all dishes. They'll make your food come alive.

Individualizing Your Diet

The starting point for the optimal Paleo Diet lies in our genes. In some respects, we're all the same. We've all got the basic human genome, shaped by more than 2 million years of evolution and adapted to eat lean, wild animal meats and uncultivated fruits and vegetables. But we're all different, too. Our own genetic differences ultimately influence how we react to certain foods or food types, or how much of a particular nutrient, vitamin, or mineral we need to maintain good health. Even though seafood should be a central part of the Paleo Diet, for example, it's clearly out of the question for people who are allergic to it. If you have a nut, shellfish, or other food allergy, then obviously these foods cannot be part of your individualized program.

The National Academy of Sciences has provided DRIs (Dietary Reference Intakes) for vitamins and minerals. However, these one-size-fits-all guidelines aren't necessarily perfect for everyone. For example, people who are exposed to extra environmental pollutants (say, cigarette smoke) have been shown to require extra antioxidant vitamins. Certain diseases and disorders are known to impair the body's ability to absorb nutrients; pregnant women and breast-feeding mothers need more nutrients than other women do.

No universal dietary recommendations apply to everybody, even though we all have the same starting point—our evolutionary past.

Many people don't even know that some foods—particularly, grains, dairy products, legumes, and yeast—are to blame for some of their health problems. They may not make the diet/health connection until they eliminate these foods and then reintroduce them. Listen to your body as you gradually return to the diet nature intended for us all. Find out what works for you and be sensible; alter your diet so that you can live with it—but remember, the further you stray from the basic principles of the diet (lean animal protein, fresh fruits, and vegetables), the less likely you'll be able to reap its health benefits.

Vitamins, Minerals, and Supplements

When we eat the foods that we're genetically programmed to eat, we won't develop nutritional deficiency diseases. As I discussed earlier, pellagra (niacin deficiency) and beriberi (vitamin B_1 deficiency) have never been found in hunter-gatherers—modern or Paleolithic. In chapter 2 I showed how the vitamins and the minerals eaten every day on the Paleo Diet—a modern Paleo diet—far exceed the RDAs in almost every category. This diet is nutrient-rich by any standard, and it provides us with everything we need to be healthy.

This does not mean that people on the Paleo Diet don't need supplements. You may choose to bolster your diet with certain supplements, including those discussed next.

Vitamin D

Except for fatty ocean fish, there is very little vitamin D in any commonly consumed natural (that is, not artificially fortified) foods. This wasn't a major problem for our Paleolithic ancestors, who spent much of their time outdoors and got all the vitamin D they needed from sunlight. Today, for most of us, sunlight exposure is a hit-or-miss proposition. This is why, to prevent rickets and other vitamin D–deficiency diseases, processed foods such as milk and margarine are fortified with vitamin D.

Do you get enough sun? ("Enough" means about fifteen minutes a day.) If you don't, and you've stopped eating margarine and milk, you should supplement your diet with this nutrient. The DRI for vitamin D is 200–600 IU (for "international units"). Because many studies have suggested a link between low vitamin D levels in the blood and a number of cancers—including breast, prostate, and colon cancers—you may want to boost your daily supplementation to 2,000 IU. However, this is not one of those "more is better" nutrients. Vitamin D is fat-soluble, which means it can accumulate in your tissues and eventually become toxic if you take too much of it. The tolerable upper limit for vitamin D in adults is 2,000 IU daily, although recent studies have challenged this value and suggest that a more accurate limit is 10,000 IU.

Here are the keys to healthy sun exposure:

- Build up sun time gradually (fifteen minutes or less at first, depending on your skin color and ability to tan).
- Never let your skin burn.
- Where it is possible, take the sun year round.
- Use sunscreens at first to prevent burning; look for sunscreens that block both ultraviolet A and ultraviolet B sunlight.
- However, because sunscreens also impair vitamin D and melanin production, as your tan develops, you can gradually reduce the level of sunscreen protection.

Antioxidants

Although our bodies are basically the same as those of our ancient ancestors, we live in a vastly different world. The pristine, unpolluted Paleolithic environment no longer exists; we are regularly exposed to numerous toxic substances that didn't exist 100 years ago. The food we eat, the air we breathe, and the water we drink contain minuscule residues of pesticides and chemical and industrial contaminants. These pollutants are inescapable; they're even found in remote parts of Antarctica and Greenland.

Nobody knows the effects of a lifetime exposure to these noxious agents. However, it's clear that a well-functioning immune system—bolstered by antioxidant vitamins and minerals—may help protect you from a variety of environmentally dependent cancers and diseases. The medical literature is overflowing with studies showing the potential of supplemental antioxidants to reduce the risk of heart disease and many cancers.

The Paleo Diet is exceptionally rich in antioxidants—even with no supplementation. It contains, on average, more than 500 milligrams of vitamin C (more than nine times the RDA), more than 25 IU of vitamin E (more than three times the RDA), and more than 140 micrograms of selenium (more than 2.5 times the RDA). Also, because this diet is loaded with fresh fruits and vegetables, it's high in beta-carotene and many other plant substances (phytochemicals) that protect against many types of cancer. But for some antioxidants, it may be beneficial to supplement your diet. These include:

- *Vitamin E:* Many of the beneficial effects of vitamin E have been shown to occur with pharmacological doses that cannot be achieved by diet alone. Because vitamin E is completely safe and has virtually no side effects, daily doses between 200 and 400 IU may provide additional disease protection.
- *Vitamin C:* Here, too, you may want to bring your daily level higher than you could reach with diet alone. Daily supplementation of 500 to 1,000 milligrams has been shown to improve immune function, lower cholesterol, and reduce the risk of some types of cancer.
- *Selenium:* Selenium may be one of our most important allies in preventing or waylaying the cancer process. In a randomized, double-blind study (the "gold standard" in medical research) of 1,312 older people, selenium doses of 200 micrograms reduced the overall incidence of cancer by 42 percent and cut cancer death rates in half. The selenium content of fruits and vegetables varies greatly, depending on how much selenium was in the soil where the produce was grown. To make sure you get ample amounts of selenium, you would do well to supplement your diet with 200 to 400 micrograms a day.

Fish Oil Capsules

Some people just don't like fish or shellfish, no matter how it's prepared. If you're one of them, I recommend that you take daily fish oil capsules. There are two active ingredients, both fatty acids, in fish oil that produce its many beneficial effects—eicosapentaenoic acid (EPA) and docosahexaenoic acid (DHA). You should try to take 1 to 2 grams of EPA and DHA daily. Depending on the brand and the size of the capsules, you will need to take about four to eight capsules per day to get sufficient EPA and DHA. Regular fish oil supplementation will decrease your risk of cancer and heart disease and may reduce certain symptoms of autoimmune diseases and inflammatory disorders.

Food Availability and Preparation Issues

One of the keys to making this diet work is ensuring that your modern Paleo food is always available. Many of us have schedules away from home or at our jobs, where it is impossible to prepare or buy fresh, unadulterated fruits, veggies, and lean meats. This means you will need to prepare some of your food at home and bring it with you. But this isn't a problem. For most people, lunch is the most common meal away from home, and "brown-bagging" lunch is the norm for many working people.

You don't have to prepare three separate Paleo meals from scratch every single day. What works best for most people is to simply double or triple the size of the evening meal and then bring the leftovers for lunch. Put parts of your salad and main dish in a sealed container that night and take them with you the next morning. Toss in a piece of fresh fruit, and you've got a terrific lunch! You can also cook two or more main dishes in the evening, use one, and immediately refrigerate the other for use later in the week.

This same principle works for your condiments (salad dressings, salsas, marinades, dips, etc.). Mix up a big batch on the weekend or in the evening, put it in a container, and store it in the refrigerator until you need it. Nothing could be simpler.

Most supermarkets now stock precut, washed salad vegetables and mixes of lettuces. Completely mixed salads (spinach, Caesar, etc.) in sealed plastic bags without added dressing are also commonly available. These packaged veggies are great for people on the go who want to eat fresh foods but don't have time to prepare them. So if time is of the essence, you can make a wonderful, healthful salad by simply opening a bag of cut, washed, and mixed salad greens. Try tossing in some cold shrimp, shredded crabmeat, and olive oil or dressing that you have made beforehand, and you've got another instant Paleo lunch.

Dining Out, Travel, and Peer Pressure

You're invited over to a close friend's house for dinner, and it's spaghetti and meatballs. That's okay, just this once. Your daughter baked you a triple-chocolate birthday cake and would be devastated if you didn't eat at least a piece. That's okay, just this once. Things happen—and a few occasional and minor dietary indiscretions won't make much difference to your overall health if you follow the diet the rest of the time. However, if these indiscretions become the rule and not the exception, you will increasingly lose the healthful benefits and weight-loss effects of the Paleo Diet.

Dining Out

How can you make the Paleo Diet work in the real world? Do the best you can. When you dine out, it can be a challenge—or downright impossible—to follow the Paleo Diet to a T. In the real world, many restaurants build their menu around most of the foods you're trying not to eat. Even though many restaurants now offer low-fat or vegetarian meals, few restaurants sponsor Paleo cuisine. In the best situations, you'll be able to stick pretty close to the Paleo Diet; in the worst cases, you may have to throw in the towel.

However, most of the time, you should be able to pull it off with just a few transgressions. The key is "triage." Assign your priorities based on urgency:

1. Your number one concern is to *get a main dish that is not a starch-based food.* Avoid pancakes for breakfast, for example, sandwiches for lunch, and pasta for dinner.
2. Try to choose lean meat or seafood, cooked in a simple manner—by baking, broiling, sautéing, roasting, poaching, or steaming—without added starches and fats.
3. Always try to get some fresh fruit or a nonstarchy vegetable at every meal.
4. Keep the meal as simple as you can; the fewer ingredients, the better.

Breakfast

Most breakfast restaurants serve fresh fruit and some form of eggs. Because fried and scrambled eggs are usually cooked with trans fat–containing margarine or shortening, order your eggs poached or hard-boiled. Or have an omelet filled with veggies—hold the cheese and skip the toast. A cup of coffee is okay. Sometimes you can find smoked salmon or fish for breakfast or shrimp-stuffed omelets; try to include healthful omega 3 fats whenever possible. A lean ham slice or pork chop or a lean breakfast steak is another option—but make sure that you also get a big bowl of fruit to balance the acid-producing protein load. Try to keep salt to a minimum (this is probably the most difficult aspect of dining out).

Lunch

Lunches are usually pretty easy, now that most restaurants offer salads, lean meats, and fish as entrées. If your salad comes with croutons, ignore them, and try to get an olive oil–based dressing. For dessert, order fresh fruit.

Dinner

Dinners out are usually fairly easy, too. Even pasta-heavy Italian restaurants usually have seafood or meat entrées. You can ask to have these dishes prepared without added flour or breading, skip the potatoes, and get a side order of steamed vegetables. Treat yourself to an occasional glass of wine with dinner. Japanese restaurants are a breeze. They almost always have fish, shellfish, or lean beef and plenty of steamed veggies; just skip the rice and the soy sauce (it's far too salty, and most soy sauces are made with wheat). Chinese restaurants can also be dealt with deftly by avoiding dishes that are rich in sugary, salty sauces, such as sweet and sour pork and deep-fried "crispy" dishes. Go with stir-fried chicken dishes or, better yet, steamed crab or fish. Use the same strategy in ordering Chinese vegetable side dishes; ask your waiter or waitress to omit any sauces and just bring fresh steamed veggies. Mexican restaurants are a bit of a challenge, but again, with careful selections you can stick pretty closely to the Paleo Diet. Once in a while, there will be no choice; you'll have to accept whatever food is available. In those cases, limit your portions.

When You Travel

You may choose to dine out, buy food and take it with you in a cooler, or buy it in supermarkets, grocery stores, and even roadside markets along the way. Fresh fruit and veggies are universally available, and they travel well in an ice-filled cooler. Try making your own beef jerky (see chapter 10); it's delicious and filling, and it tastes great with fresh fruit. Hard-boiled eggs, cooked beforehand and stored in the cooler, can be indispensable for breakfasts on the road.

Instead of stopping where most traveling Americans do—at the first exit with a fast-food restaurant that looks fairly clean—drive a mile or two from the highway and find a supermarket. Most food stores have deli sections with premade salads, and many offer a salad bar. Apply the triage principle and do the best you can. For example, precooked chicken (roasted or rotisserie-cooked) is available at most supermarket deli counters and is an option in a pinch. Make sure to take the skin off before you eat it. If you didn't bring any paper plates and plastic utensils, pick some up while you're at the store. Water-packed tuna isn't ideal, either, but it will do while you're on the road.

Ask Your Friends and Family for Support

The support of your spouse, immediate family, and friends can make a world of difference in any big life change. Tell them what you're doing and why—whether it's to lose weight or to improve your health. Explain the logic and rationale of the Paleo Diet and share your successes with them. You don't necessarily have to put the entire family on the diet, and many of the meals that you'll be eating on this lifetime program of nutrition are not very different from the types of food you ate before. You can always include bread, rolls, or potatoes with your family meals and give family members the option of eating them. In nearly all public settings, unless you call it to their attention, most people won't even realize that your diet has changed—until they notice your weight loss, increase in energy level, and improvement in health. Who knows? They may see the healthful changes you're experiencing and want to join you.

The Paleo Diet is humanity's *normal* diet. The abnormal diet, the odd diet, the out-of-the-ordinary diet is actually the grain-, dairy-, and processed food–based diet that currently pervades the Western world. It's time for a change.

9

The Meal Plans
for the Three Levels
of the Paleo Diet

The Paleo Diet is a lifelong way of eating that will gradually restore your normal body weight, health, and well-being. If you follow the dietary guidelines and principles I have laid out, you will reap all the benefits that humanity's original diet has to offer. Your health will immediately improve, and you will definitely begin to lose weight.

In this chapter, you'll find three two-week meal plans. Any of them will work for you; the only difference is in the number of Open Meals. Level I allows you three Open Meals per week, Level II allows two per week, and Level III allows one. Just use the appropriate number of Open Meals for your level of the diet, and you're set. Use these guidelines and the recipes in chapter 10 to help you embrace the diet that nature designed for us all.

If you are a beginner, you may want to adhere to Level I for two to four weeks before you move to Levels II and III—or, if you're happy there, you may want to stay at this level of the diet. Note: You should try to include no more than one Open Meal on any given day, and do not try to make up for lost time with your meal choices. Use them as a safety net as you get used to humanity's *real* foods: fresh, lean meats, seafood, and fruits and vegetables.

Should you definitely plan to move up to Levels II and III? Not necessarily. Depending on your nutritional and weight-loss goals, .

you may be happy with the results you achieve at Level I, particularly if you limit your consumption of the non-Paleo foods while consuming your Open Meals.

If you decide to jump into the Paleo Diet more rapidly by advancing to Level II, then you may substitute two Open Meals a week for any of the meals in the meal plans.

If you are one of those people who can make long-term behavioral changes abruptly and want to go cold turkey to the Stone Age, or if it is absolutely essential that you maximize the weight-loss and health benefits of this program, then you should adopt Level III. On Level III you should substitute one Open Meal a week for any of the meal plans.

However, most people do quite well at Level II, and this is the level I recommend for maintenance, except for dieters with chronic diseases, who may do better with long-term adherence to Level III.

Snacks

When our ancient ancestors were out foraging for food, they often snacked on some of the food they gathered, or they took portions of a previous meal along their journey. The snacks on the Paleo Diet—like those of our Paleo ancestors—are healthy, wholesome, and made of real food. Most of them are easily portable, so you may want to bring some of them along on your own daily journeys. You may eat snacks between meals whenever you become hungry.

- Fresh fruit of any kind
- Homemade beef jerky (without salt)
- Homemade dried salmon strips (without salt)
- Raw vegetables: carrots, celery sticks, cherry tomatoes, mushrooms, broccoli, cucumbers, cauliflower (with homemade guacamole or salsa dip)
- Cold skinless, broiled chicken breast
- Avocado or tomato slices
- Nuts: almonds, pecans, walnuts, filberts (limit to 4 ounces a day if you're trying to lose weight)
- Dried fruit (limit to 2 ounces a day)
- Hard-boiled egg
- Cold slices of lean beef
- Peel-and-eat shrimp

- Unsalted sunflower seeds (limit to 4 ounces a day if you're trying to lose weight)

Level I: Entry Level

The key to Level I is the 85-15 rule, and here's how it works: Most people eat about twenty meals a week, plus snacks. On this beginning level, three of your meals—15 percent of the meals you eat all week—can be "open." This way, you don't have to give up your favorite foods. Again, the flexibility of the Paleo Diet allows you to cheat occasionally without losing the overall benefits of the diet. The three Open Meals provide a good opportunity to taste some of the foods you may miss the most.

There is great potential for abuse here, and you should do your best to avoid it. Do not consider these Open Meals as your chance to pig out on forbidden foods. For example, having two pints of Ben & Jerry's Chunky Monkey ice cream for lunch would be a bad move and self-defeating. But if you're invited to a party or go out to eat with friends, the Open Meal is your chance to indulge a bit. A single scoop of Chunky Monkey won't hurt, particularly if you've been on the diet all week. Or eat a slice of toast with your breakfast or have some potatoes with your dinner entrée. But again, don't eat six slices of toast or a pound of mashed potatoes. The basic idea is to ease the feeling of deprivation that generally accompanies the start of any change in diet. If you handle these Open Meals wisely—treating yourself, but not to excess—you'll soon find that you don't need to cheat at all.

At first, many people find it difficult to give up bread, cereals, and dairy products. But when you cut down on these foods gradually, you'll eventually be able to replace them with more healthful fruits and vegetables. With Level I, you may want to use some "transitional" condiments. These contain sugar and salt but are low in fat. As you become accustomed to your new eating plan, you'll want to reduce or eliminate them. Transitional condiments include:

- Low-fat salad dressings. Use these in moderation and read the labels. Stay away from brands that contain large amounts of corn syrup or salt.
- Commercial sauces. Mustard, hot sauces, prepared salsa. Note: *No catsup* (except for the Paleo version, the recipe for

which is included in chapter 10); regular catsup is too high
in salt and fructose.

If you are a coffee, beer, or wine drinker, you may continue to
enjoy these non-Paleo beverages in moderation, working toward
cutting back on them as you become accustomed to the Paleo
Diet. Transitional beverages include:

- Sugar-free soft drinks. Use these in moderation. All of them
  contain artificial sweeteners, which are best left out of your
  diet.
- Alcoholic beverages. Use these in moderation.
- Coffee. Use it in moderation. Excessive caffeine is associated
  with a number of illnesses and health problems.

Sample Two-Week Meal Plan for Level I

SUNDAY   *Breakfast:* Open
                Lunch:
                    Almond Chicken Salad*
                    Herbal tea
                Dinner:
                    Tomato and avocado slices
                    Grilled skinless turkey breast
                    Steamed broccoli, carrots, and artichoke
                    Bowl of fresh blueberries, raisins, and almonds
                    Water with lemon slice
                Snack: Basic Beef Jerky,* celery sticks

MONDAY   *Breakfast:*
                    Bowl of diced apples, shredded carrots, and raisins
                    Poached eggs
                    Cup of decaffeinated coffee
                Lunch:
                    Brockway Tuna Salad*
                    Handful of almonds
                    Mineral water
                Dinner:
                    Escargots (prepared without butter)
                    Tossed green salad
                    Broiled halibut steak with lemon juice and dill

---

* See recipes in chapter 10.

Steamed asparagus
Sliced kiwi fruit and tangerine wedges
Glass of dry white wine
Snack: cold lean beef slices, carrot sticks

TUESDAY   *Breakfast:*
Cantaloupe, strawberries
Broiled lean pork chops
Herbal tea
Lunch:
Spinach salad with choice of Paleo dressing*
Broiled orange roughy with fresh orange juice
    and oregano
Steamed cauliflower
Apple
Mineral water
Dinner:
Paleo Zucchini Soup*
Slow-Cooked Veal with Salsa*
Figs
Iced tea
Snack: hard-boiled eggs, walnuts, raisins

WEDNESDAY   *Breakfast:*
Grapefruit
Strawberries with blackberries
Cold leftover Veal with Salsa*
Cup of decaffeinated coffee
Lunch: Open
Dinner:
Avocado and tomato slices
Oysters on the half shell
Altamira Stuffed Chicken*
Ratatouille*
Fresh boysenberries, raisins, and almonds
Cup of decaffeinated coffee
Snack: mango, unsalted macadamia nuts,
Dried Salmon*

THURSDAY   *Breakfast:*
Raspberries with walnuts
Scrambled eggs with a small beefsteak
Herbal tea

Lunch:
    Lime and Dill Crab*
    Figs and fresh nectarines
    Iced tea
Dinner:
    Spicy Tomato Soup*
    Green salad with black olives (rinsed of salt)
    Burgundy Walnut Beef Roast*
    Steamed cauliflower with lemon juice and paprika
    Fresh peaches
    Glass of red wine
Snack: cold chicken breast, cherry tomatoes,
    celery sticks

FRIDAY   *Breakfast:*
    Blueberries and cantaloupe
    Cold crab legs
    Water with lemon
Lunch:
    Gingery Chicken and Veggies*
    Tomato/black olive (rinsed of salt), green salad,
        and Anaheim Cilantro Salsa* dressing
    Iced tea
Dinner: Open
Snack: hard-boiled eggs, cold broiled salmon steak

SATURDAY   *Breakfast:*
    Casaba melon
    Cold chicken breasts
    Herbal tea
Lunch:
    Tahoe Shrimp Salad*
    Melon slices and strawberries
    Sugar-free soda
Dinner:
    Cold mackerel
    Tomato and cucumber wedges with olive oil
        and lemon juice
    Auroch Beef Cabbage Rolls*
    Chopped pecans, raspberries, and Medjool dates
    Water with lemon wedge
Snack: Basic Beef Jerky,* apple slices

SUNDAY   *Breakfast:*
               Bowl of sliced bananas, strawberries, and walnuts
               Cup of decaffeinated coffee
           Lunch:
               Waldorf Salad*
               Apple
               Water and lemon juice
           Dinner: Open
           Snack: Guava, dried apricots, kiwi fruit,
               Dried Salmon*

MONDAY   *Breakfast:*
               Cantaloupe Stuffed with Blackberries and Pecans*
               Herbal tea
           Lunch:
               Spinach Salad à la Cordani*
               Orange sections
               Mineral water
           Dinner:
               Chicken Vegetable Soup*
               Marinated Mushrooms*
               Omega Meatballs*
               Baked Walnut-Cinnamon Apples*
               Iced tea
           Snack: Spicy Beef Jerky,* dried apricots without
               sulfur

TUESDAY   *Breakfast:*
               Fresh or frozen blackberries and raspberries
               Trout sautéed in olive oil and lemon juice
               Water with lemon wedge
           Lunch:
               Turkey burgers
               Tossed green salad with olive oil and lemon juice
               Apple slices with lemon juice and mint leaves
               Iced tea
           Dinner:
               Tossed green salad with flaxseed oil and
                 lemon juice
               Paleo Zucchini Soup*
               Baked Tomatoes*
               Savory Steamed Mussels*

Fresh melon

Mineral water

Snack: fresh peaches, peel-and-eat shrimp, walnuts

WEDNESDAY *Breakfast:*

Fresh or frozen strawberries and/or blueberries

Grilled lean venison sausage

Herbal tea

Lunch: Open

Dinner:

Celery and carrot sticks dipped in Guacamole
    Fiesta*

Spicy Tomato Soup*

Steamed asparagus

Sautéed Rocky Mountain Chicken Livers*

Pomegranate

Cup of decaffeinated coffee

Snack: hard-boiled egg, unsalted macadamia nuts

THURSDAY *Breakfast:*

Fresh plums

Small lean beefsteak covered with Peach Salsa*

Cup of decaffeinated coffee

Lunch:

Gazpacho*

Shrimp-Stuffed Avocado*

Apple

Iced tea

Dinner:

Tomato, cucumber, and red onion salad with
    olive oil

Red Snapper in Snappy Sauce*

Carrot-Mushroom Stir-Fry*

Peach-Almond Delight*

Glass of dry white wine or mineral water

Snack: cold crab legs, tomato quarters

FRIDAY *Breakfast:*

Grapefruit

Scrambled Basil Eggs Topped with Salsa*

Herbal tea

Lunch:
    Tossed green salad with olive oil and lemon
      juice
    Paleo-Correct Meat Loaf*
    Glass of lemon water
Dinner:
    Marinated Mushrooms*
    Altamira Stuffed Chicken*
    Spicy Stuffed Squash*
    Baked Walnut-Cinnamon Apples*
    Mineral water
Snack: sliced cold turkey breasts, sunflower seeds,
    hard-boiled eggs

SATURDAY   *Breakfast:* Open
Lunch:
    Broiled Tenderloin of Pork with Spicy Rub*
    Honeydew melon
    Herbal tea
Dinner:
    Waldorf Salad*
    Chicken Cacciatore*
    Steamed broccoli with lemon juice
    2 or 3 Medjool dates
    Diet soda
Snack: carrot and celery sticks, dried pears,
    walnuts

Level II: Maintenance Level

Level II of the Paleo Diet is structured around the 90-10 split. Two Open Meals are permitted each week; the rest of your meals are made up of modern Paleo foods. At this level, you should restrict or eliminate all of the transitional foods, except during your two Open Meals. As in Level I, all snacks should be chosen from the list of Paleo snacks (see "snacks" near the beginning of this chapter). Many people do quite well at this level and find that there's no need to move to the next level unless weight loss or health considerations are paramount.

Sample Two-Week Meal Plan for Level II

SUNDAY   *Breakfast:* Open
               Lunch:
                  Beef and Spinach Scramble*
                  Herbal tea
               Dinner:
                  Tomato wedges and cucumber slices dipped
                      in flaxseed oil
                  Salmon Steaks in Curry Sauce*
                  Steamed brussels sprouts
                  Tangerines
                  Mineral water
               Snack: apple with Spicy Beef Jerky*

MONDAY   *Breakfast:*
                  Half a cantaloupe, strawberries
                  Cold halibut steak
                  Herbal tea
               Lunch:
                  Brockway Tuna Salad*
                  Tangerine
                  Water with lemon
               Dinner:
                  Tomato and cucumber slices with Veggie Dip*
                  Omega Meatballs*
                  Steamed carrots and cauliflower with dill and
                      paprika
                  Kiwi fruit and strawberries with walnut pieces
                  Iced herbal tea
               Snack: Spicy Beef Jerky,* celery sticks

TUESDAY   *Breakfast:*
                  Grapefruit
                  Two-egg (omega 3–enriched) omelet with
                      avocado, scallion, and tomato filling cooked
                      in olive oil
                  Herbal tea
               Lunch:
                  Gingery Chicken and Veggies*
                  Apple and walnuts
                  Diet soda

Dinner:
>Tomato wedges
>Artichoke leaves dipped in Omega 3 Mayonnaise*
>Tossed green salad with flaxseed oil and lemon
>>juice
>Salmon Steaks in Curry Sauce*
>Fresh or frozen berries
>Glass of nonalcoholic wine

Snack: carrot sticks, sliced zucchini, cold boiled shrimp

WEDNESDAY   *Breakfast:* Open
Lunch:
>Gazpacho*
>Cajun Catfish Bake*
>Fresh peaches
>Herbal tea

Dinner:
>Chicken Vegetable Soup*
>Ambrosia Salad*
>Barbecued Alaskan Shrimp*
>Fresh blackberries
>Glass of ice water and lemon wedge

Snack: walnuts and raisins, hard-boiled egg

THURSDAY   *Breakfast:*
>Fresh pineapple slices
>Broiled small breakfast steak covered with
>>Anaheim Cilantro Salsa*
>Herbal tea

Lunch:
>Spinach Salad with Crabmeat*
>Fresh oranges
>Mineral water

Dinner:
>Butter Leaf Avocado Salad*
>Baked Haddock Italiano*
>Steamed summer squash with lemon pepper
>>and paprika
>Fresh Cinnamon Applesauce*
>Water with lemon slice

Snack: cold chicken breasts, celery and carrot sticks

FRIDAY   *Breakfast:*
    Pink grapefruit
    Chilled steamed prawns
    Cup of decaffeinated coffee
Lunch:
    Tossed green salad with Omega 3 Russian
        Dressing*
    Grilled lean pork chops covered with Raspberry
        Barbecue Sauce*
    Mineral water
Dinner: Open
Snack: cucumber slices, cold lean beef slices

SATURDAY   *Breakfast:*
    Fresh or frozen strawberries
    Two-egg (omega 3–enriched) omelet stuffed
        with spinach, mushrooms, and onions sautéed
        in olive oil
    Water with fresh lemon wedge
Lunch:
    Kenny's Barbecued Spicy Chicken*
    Steamed vegetables
    Fresh fruit
    Diet soda
Dinner:
    Marinated Mushrooms*
    Red Snapper in Snappy Sauce*
    Spicy Stuffed Squash*
    Baked Walnut-Cinnamon Apples*
    Glass of Sancerre wine
Snack: Basic Beef Jerky,* dried apple slices

SUNDAY   *Breakfast:*
    Honeydew melon and fresh blueberries covered
        with walnuts
    Chilled steamed crab legs
    Cup of decaffeinated coffee
Lunch:
    Tossed green salad with Omega 3 Russian Salad
        Dressing*
    Broiled flounder with lemon juice and dill
    Glass of nonalcoholic cabernet sauvignon wine

Dinner:
Tomato and avocado wedges with garlic and
    cayenne powders
Sicilian Skillet Veal Chops*
Steamed cauliflower served with lemon juice
Carrot sticks
Strawberry-Blueberry Horizon*
Iced herbal tea
Snack: celery and carrot sticks dipped in Veggie
    Dip,* unsalted macadamia nuts

MONDAY   *Breakfast:*
Kyle's Apple Breakfast*
Cold sliced turkey breast
Herbal tea
Lunch:
Auroch Beef Cabbage Rolls*
Fresh fruit
Iced herbal tea
Dinner:
Gazpacho*
Mackerel steaks with dill and lemon juice
Steamed asparagus with lemon juice
Fresh fruit
Glass of nonalcoholic wine
Snack: Spicy Beef Jerky,* dried apricots without sulfur

TUESDAY   *Breakfast:*
Fresh orange slices
Scrambled Basil Eggs Topped with Salsa*
Cup of decaffeinated coffee
Lunch:
Carrot Salad*
Salmon Steaks in Curry Sauce*
Mineral water
Dinner:
Baked Tomatoes*
Rocky Mountain Elk Steaks*
Walnut Broccoli with Carrots*
Almost Frozen Mashed Bananas*
Ice water
Snack: Dried Salmon,* kiwi fruit, celery sticks

WEDNESDAY   *Breakfast:*
            Fresh papaya
            Pork Chops Stuffed with Chicken Livers*
            Ice water with lime wedge
            Lunch: Open
            Dinner:
            Tossed green salad with olive oil and lemon
                juice
            Burgundy Walnut Beef Roast*
            Steamed orange peppers and onions
            Peach-Almond Delight*
            Iced tea
            Snack: cold trout, slices of Vidalia or Maui sweet
            onions, oranges

THURSDAY   *Breakfast:*
            Grapefruit
            Cold beef slices
            Cup of decaffeinated coffee
            Lunch:
            Spinach salad with shrimp
            Apple slices with lemon juice
            Herbal tea
            Dinner:
            Tossed green salad dressed with flaxseed oil
                and lemon juice
            Paleo Zucchini Soup*
            Broiled chicken breasts covered with Peach
                Salsa*
            Fresh Cinnamon Applesauce*
            Iced tea
            Snack: walnuts, grapes, cherry tomatoes

FRIDAY   *Breakfast:*
            Cantaloupe
            Poached Eggs with Peach Salsa*
            Herbal tea
            Lunch:
            Tossed green salad with Omega 3 Russian Dressing*
            Lime and Dill Crab*
            Steamed carrots
            Water with lemon wedge

Dinner:
>   Chicken Vegetable Soup*
>   Paleo-Correct Meat Loaf*
>   Avocado and tomato slices
>   Steamed broccoli
>   Fresh peaches
>   Glass of Pinot Noir wine

Snack: Peel-and-eat shrimp, celery sticks, pecans

SATURDAY   *Breakfast:*
>   Citrus bowl (grapefruit, orange, and tangerine
>   sections)
>   Cold Paleo-Correct Meat Loaf* (left over from
>   dinner)
>   Herbal tea

Lunch:
>   Tomato, cucumber, purple onion salad with
>   olive oil
>   Beef and Spinach Scramble*
>   Mineral water

Dinner:
>   Sliced cucumber and radish tray
>   Chez Lorraine's Baked Salmon*
>   Steamed asparagus
>   Pecans, raisins, and blueberries
>   Cup of decaffeinated coffee

Snack: cold chicken breasts, sunflower seeds,
>   dried pear slices

Level III: Maximal Weight Loss Level

At Level III, it's the 95-5 rule—with one Open Meal a week, and the balance of meals made up of all the delicious modern Paleo meals I've discussed in this chapter. At this level, you should restrict or eliminate all the transitional foods, except during your Open Meals. As in Levels I and II, all snacks should be chosen from the list of Paleo Snacks. This is the highest level, designed for the true Paleo Diet aficionado who wants to maximize health and well-being, or for individuals suffering from actual obesity or high levels of chronic disease who need to maximize the therapeutic effects of the diet.

Sample Two-Week Meal Plan for Level III

SUNDAY   *Breakfast:* Open
                Lunch:
                      Tossed green salad with lemon juice and
                          olive oil dressing
                      Savory Steamed Mussels*
                      Mineral water
                Dinner:
                      Tomato and avocado slices
                      Altamira Stuffed Chicken*
                      Steamed Swiss chard and carrots
                      Steamed artichoke
                      Bowl of fresh blueberries, raisins, and almonds
                      Mineral water
                Snack: Basic Beef Jerky,* carrot sticks

MONDAY   *Breakfast:*
                      Bowl of diced apples, shredded carrots, and
                          raisins with cinnamon
                      Poached eggs
                      Cup of decaffeinated coffee
                Lunch:
                      Brockway Tuna Salad*
                      Handful of walnuts
                      Mineral water
                Dinner:
                      Peel-and-eat shrimp
                      Tossed green salad
                      Chez Lorraine's Baked Salmon*
                      Steamed asparagus with fresh-squeezed lemon
                      Sliced kiwi fruit and strawberries
                      Diet soda
                Snack: cold lean beef slices, celery sticks

TUESDAY   *Breakfast:*
                      Honeydew melon, blackberries
                      Broiled lean pork chops
                      Herbal tea
                Lunch:
                      Waldorf Salad*
                      Broiled halibut steak with lime juice
                      Steamed cauliflower

Apple

Mineral water

Dinner:

Tossed green salad with scallions and
cucumbers

Chicken Vegetable Soup*

Stir-Fried Beef with Vegetables*

Figs and walnuts

Iced tea

Snack: hard-boiled eggs, pecans, raisins

WEDNESDAY   *Breakfast:*

Strawberries and apricots

Zesty Shrimp-Avocado Omelet*

Cup of decaffeinated coffee

Lunch:

Cucumber and tomato slices with Veggie Dip*

Steamed crab

Dried apricots

Mineral water

Dinner:

Oysters on the half shell

Cucumber slices dipped in Guacamole Fiesta*

Altamira Stuffed Chicken*

Ratatouille*

Bowl of fresh boysenberries, raisins, and almonds

Glass of nonalcoholic dry white wine

Snack: papaya, walnuts, Spicy Beef Jerky*

THURSDAY   *Breakfast:*

Strawberries

Small beefsteak with Peach Salsa*

Herbal tea

Lunch:

Tossed green salad with flaxseed oil and lemon
juice

Sand Harbor Baked Cod*

Medjool dates and fresh nectarines

Iced tea

Dinner:

Marinated Mushrooms*

Green salad with olive oil and lemon juice

Broiled Tenderloin of Pork with Spicy Rub*
Steamed cabbage with lemon juice and paprika
Baked Walnut-Cinnamon Apples*
Glass of ice water
Snack: cold chicken breast, cantaloupe

FRIDAY   *Breakfast:*
Fresh or frozen blueberries and cantaloupe
Cold steamed king crab legs
Water with lemon
Lunch:
Green salad with avocado, quartered tomatoes,
    and black olives (rinsed of salt) dressed with
    Anaheim Cilantro Salsa*
Gingery Chicken and Veggies*
Apple
Mineral water
Dinner:
Spinach salad with walnuts and flaxseed oil
    dressing
Cold trout
Baked Tomatoes*
Chopped pecans, raspberries, and Medjool dates
Mineral water
Snack: hard-boiled egg, cold prawns

SATURDAY   *Breakfast:*
Cold chicken breasts covered with Anaheim
    Cilantro Salsa*
Watermelon
Herbal tea
Lunch:
Tahoe Shrimp Salad*
Melon slices and strawberries
Sugar-free Diet 7-Up
Dinner:
Carrot, radish, cherry tomato, sliced cucumber tray
Baked Haddock Italiano*
Steamed asparagus
Almonds, raisins, and peaches
Mineral water
Snack: Basic Beef Jerky,* oranges

SUNDAY   *Breakfast:*
    Bowl of sliced banana, pears, walnuts
    Soft-boiled eggs
    Cup of decaffeinated coffee
  Lunch:
    Tossed green salad dressed with olive oil
        and lemon juice
    Red Snapper in Snappy Sauce*
    Apple slices with lemon juice
    Mineral water
  Dinner:
    Ambrosia Salad*
    Broiled lobster tails with olive oil and fresh pepper
    Steamed artichoke with lemon juice
    Strawberry-Blueberry Horizon*
    Cup of decaffeinated coffee
  Snack: mango, kiwi fruit, Dried Salmon*

MONDAY   *Breakfast:*
    Cantaloupe Stuffed with Blackberries and Pecans*
    Cold leftover lobster
    Herbal tea
  Lunch:
    Tossed green salad with olive oil and lemon juice
    Kenny's Barbecued Spicy Chicken*
    Tangerine sections
    Glass of nonalcoholic chardonnay
  Dinner:
    Marinated Mushrooms*
    Chicken Vegetable Soup*
    London broil sprinkled with fresh ground
      pepper and garlic powder
    Spicy Stuffed Squash*
    Peach-Almond Delight*
    Iced tea
  Snack: Kyle's Apple Breakfast,* Spicy Beef
    Jerky*

TUESDAY   *Breakfast:*
    Grapefruit
    Cold leftover London broil
    Herbal tea

Lunch:
> Gazpacho*
> Broiled turkey burgers
> Sliced star fruit
> Mineral water

Dinner:
> Butter Leaf Avocado Salad*
> Cajun Catfish Bake*
> Steamed collard greens
> Cantaloupe Stuffed with Blackberries and Pecans*
> Glass of mineral water

Snack: peel-and-eat shrimp, cauliflower florets, pecans

WEDNESDAY   *Breakfast:*
> Fresh mangos and papayas
> Lean breakfast beefsteak smothered with Peach Salsa*
> Herbal tea

Lunch:
> Celery and carrot sticks dipped in Guacamole Fiesta*
> Paleo Zucchini Soup*
> Sautéed Rocky Mountain Chicken Livers*
> Fresh blueberries
> Water with lemon slice

Dinner:
> Spinach Salad à la Cordani*
> Tender Buffalo Roast*
> Steamed asparagus and carrots with lemon juice and garlic powder
> Fresh Cinnamon Applesauce*
> Cup of decaffeinated coffee

Snack: hard-boiled egg, walnuts, raisins

THURSDAY   *Breakfast:*
> Fresh plums
> Cold leftover Tender Buffalo Roast* slices covered with fresh Anaheim Cilantro Salsa*
> Lemon water

Lunch:
> Spicy Tomato Soup*

Shrimp-Stuffed Avocado*
Watermelon
Diet soda

Dinner:
Tomato, cucumber, and purple onion salad
    with olive oil
Roast Pheasant with Fruit and Nut Stuffing*
Carrot-Mushroom Stir-Fry*
Waldorf Salad*
Glass of red wine or mineral water
Snack: cold, lean steak slices; tomato quarters

FRIDAY *Breakfast:*
Cantaloupe
Eggs scrambled in olive oil and basil
Herbal tea

Lunch:
Almond Chicken Salad*
Glass of lemon water

Dinner:
Marinated Mushrooms*
Isola Baked Pork Chops*
Ratatouille*
Baked Walnut-Cinnamon Apples*
Diet soda
Snack: cold chicken breasts, sunflower seeds

SATURDAY *Breakfast:*
Fresh or frozen strawberries
Poached eggs, cold prawns
Tea

Lunch: Open

Dinner:
Tossed green salad with flaxseed oil and
    lemon juice
Barbecued Venison Steaks with Herbs*
Steamed summer squash with lemon
    juice
Walnut Broccoli with Carrots*
2 or 3 Medjool dates
Ice water
Snack: carrot and celery sticks, raisins, walnuts

So there you have it—three delicious and healthful meal plans (Level I: three Open Meals per week; Level II: two Open Meals per week; and Level III: one Open Meal per week). Use these meal plans to familiarize yourself with Paleo Diet principles. Once you have become a seasoned Paleo Dieter, use your own creativity and ingenuity to develop your own scrumptious Paleo feasts!

10

Paleo Recipes

With the Paleo Diet, you'll end up eating enormously diverse and bountiful meals that include all sorts of fruits, vegetables, meats, and seafood—many of which are rarely or never eaten on "normal" diets.

Throughout this book, I've been telling you how good this food is. In this chapter, I'm going to prove it. On the following pages you'll find a wide variety of breakfast, lunch, and dinner recipes, as well as recipes for making Stone Age snacks and desserts, salt- and sugar-free sauces, dressings, salsas, and condiments to help you launch the Paleo Diet in your own kitchen. Consider them a starting point for your own creativity and ingenuity. Starting the Paleo Diet doesn't mean you'll have to throw out your old cookbooks. It is easy to modify almost any basic recipe to conform to Stone Age dietary principles. I've also just published *The Paleo Diet Cookbook*, which contains more than 150 recipes not found in this revised edition of the diet plan.

One cautionary note: In all your cooking, do your best to follow the spirit of the diet. If you eat certain Paleo foods or food combinations excessively, you can sabotage and defeat this lifetime nutrition plan and even gain weight. With modern food-processing techniques and creative recipes, a clever cook can assemble Stone Age ingredients in a manner that defies the basic logic of the diet. For instance, it is possible to make nut and root flours in food processors that can be combined with honey, olive oil, and eggs and later baked to resemble almost any modern processed food with very un-Paleo characteristics—high in carbohydrates, sugar, and fats. Those high-fat, high-sugar, high-carbohydrate Paleo food combinations may taste good, but they're not much better for your health and well-being than cookies, cakes, breads, and doughnuts. These foods are great treats to be eaten every once in a while and are better for you than the commercially available, processed versions. But if they become common fare—particularly if you're trying to lose weight—many of the potential benefits of the Paleo Diet will be lost.

When eaten in excessive quantities, even unprocessed or minimally processed foods that would have been available to our Paleolithic ancestors, such as dried fruits (raisins, dates, figs, and others), nuts, and honey, can throw the diet off balance and can be particularly troublesome if you're trying to lose weight. The best way to satisfy your craving for sweets is to eat fresh fruit. Instead of pie, think melons—or blueberries, blackberries, pears, peaches, strawberries, or any other favorite fresh fruit.

If you still feel hungry after eating a Paleo meal, eat more lean protein—chicken or turkey breasts, fish, lean beef, shrimp, crab, or game meat if you can get it—or more crisp, succulent vegetables or juicy, sweet, fresh fruit.

When you carefully examine the Paleo Diet recipes, you'll notice that most of them contain only fresh meats, seafood, fruits, vegetables, nuts, and seeds, with added spices, certain oils, and condiments made from all of these ingredients. Stick to these foods. Depending on your level of the Paleo Diet (I, II, or III), you may occasionally want to include a few recipes that contain vinegar, wine, honey, or a dash of salt. There's nothing wrong with eating these foods *occasionally*, unless you have a health problem or an autoimmune disease, as discussed earlier in the book. Enjoy a glass of wine, a trace of salt in your food, a bit of honey in your dessert, or even an occasional bagel—but don't make them your norm.

Basic Recipe Principles

When you make Paleo recipes with modern foods, make sure that all the ingredients are free of:

- grains
- legumes, including peanuts
- dairy products

- salt
- yeast (baked goods, pickled foods, vinegar, fermented foods, and fermented beverages all contain yeast, which may cause trouble for people with autoimmune diseases)
- processed sugars
- potatoes
- added fats (except for permitted oils in limited quantities)

Try to choose lean cuts of domestic meats. Cook simply by baking, broiling, steaming, or sautéeing in a little oil.

Stone Age Food Substitutions

Salt

Substitute powdered garlic, powdered onion, lemon juice, lime juice, lemon crystals, lemon pepper free of salt, cayenne pepper, chili powder, commercially available salt-free spice mixes, black pepper, cumin, turmeric, ground cloves, oregano, ground allspice, celery seeds, coriander seeds, and ground cardamom seeds. Actually, any spice or combination of spices can be used to replace salt. I do not recommend using any of the so-called lite salts or potassium chloride salts, because chloride, like sodium, is not good for your health.

Vinegar

Substitute lemon or lime juice (fresh or reconstituted). For tomato-containing recipes such as salsa, replace vinegar with lime juice; with fruit recipes, lemon juice usually works.

Butter/Fat

Replace butter, margarine, shortening, or lard with olive oil, flaxseed oil, walnut oil, or avocado oil. As I've discussed, olive oil has a wonderful flavor and is high in the health-promoting mono-unsaturated fats but generally has a poor omega 6 to omega 3 fat ratio. The same holds true for avocado oil. These two oils should frequently be complemented by, or blended with, other oils containing better omega 6 to omega 3 ratios such as flaxseed or walnut oils. The only oil you should cook with is olive oil. Flaxseed and walnut oils are unstable during cooking and may produce toxic by-products.

Sugars

Concentrated sugars of any kind—even natural sugars (honey, maple sugar, and date sugar)—were not staple components for our Paleolithic ancestors. Sugars in the Paleo Diet should be obtained mainly from fruits and vegetables, not from concentrated sources. However, fruit purees flavored with lemon juice and spices (cinnamon, nutmeg, mint leaves, ginger, and vanilla, to name a few) can be used in recipes to add sweetness to sauces, condiments, and desserts.

Alcohol

Alcoholic beverages clearly were not a component of true Paleolithic diets, and yours should be limited to an occasional glass of wine, beer, or spirits as part of your Open Meals. Wine, as long as it does not contain salt (as most cooking wines do), can be used to marinate meats and add flavor to many cooked dishes. When wine is used in this context, the amount of added alcohol and sugar is negligible; also, wine contains a number of health-promoting phytochemicals and antioxidants. Note: If you suffer from an autoimmune disease, the alcohol and the yeast in wine or other alcoholic beverages can potentially cause problems, and you would be wise to avoid them altogether.

Cereals

Nut flours (almond, pecan, walnut, hazelnut) can be made in food processors or purchased at some health food or specialty stores, and they can be used to thicken sauces or to add flavor to condiments. Again, these products should be used sparingly. They have the potential to unbalance your diet and disrupt your health when they're used excessively or in combination with oils, honey, dried fruit, or fruit purees. The foundation of Paleo Diet carbohydrates is fresh fruits and vegetables—not nut flours, honey, fruit juices, or purees.

Now, *bon appetit*!

Recipes

Many thanks to Don Wiss, Patti Vincent, and all of the other cooks, Paleochefs, gourmets, and gourmands at PaleoFood.com for inspiring me.

FISH AND SEAFOOD

Cajun Catfish Bake

2 lb catfish
4 T olive oil
1 clove garlic, minced
3 T freshly squeezed lemon juice

1½ tsp black pepper
½ tsp cayenne pepper
½ tsp turmeric

Thoroughly wash catfish and place in a 9 × 13-inch baking dish greased with a little olive oil. Heat the rest of the olive oil in a saucepan and sauté garlic. Pour over catfish. Sprinkle lemon juice and remaining spices evenly over fish. Bake at 350 degrees for twenty to twenty-five minutes. Serves three to four.

Sand Harbor Baked Cod

1 lb cod filets
½ c white wine
¼ yellow onion, sliced

2 T lemon juice
1 T dried dill
1 tsp turmeric

Wash fish thoroughly in cool water, and lay it in a shallow baking dish. Pour in white wine. Spread onion slices evenly over fish, and sprinkle with lemon juice, dill, and turmeric. Cover with foil, and bake at 375 degrees for twenty minutes or until fish flakes easily with a fork. Serves two to three.

Lime and Dill Crab

2 large Dungeness crabs,
   cooked, cracked, shelled,
   and chilled
2 T lime juice

2 tsp paprika
2 tsp dried, ground dill weed
2–3 limes, cut into wedges
3–4 sprigs parsley, finely chopped

Drizzle crabmeat with lime juice and sprinkle with paprika and dill. Serve with lime wedges and garnish with parsley. Serves two.

Baked Haddock Italiano

2 lb haddock
6 T olive oil
3 cloves garlic, minced
1 red onion, minced
1 green pepper, chopped
4 tomatoes, diced

6 T fresh chopped parsley
1 tsp dried basil
1 tsp dill weed
⅛ tsp black pepper
2 T lemon juice

Thoroughly wash haddock in cool water and set aside. Heat oil in a heavy skillet, and sauté garlic and onion until tender. Add green peppers and continue to sauté on low heat until tender. Add tomatoes, parsley, basil, dill, and black pepper. Remove from heat and spread half the sauce in the bottom of a 9 × 13-inch baking dish. Place fish on top, and pour remaining sauce over entire fish. Sprinkle with lemon juice. Cover with foil, and bake at 375 degrees for fifteen to twenty minutes or until flaky. Serves four.

Savory Steamed Mussels

1 lb fresh mussels in shells
½ c water
1 clove garlic, minced
2 T olive oil

1 tsp dill
1 T fresh lemon juice
½ c dry white wine

Steam mussels in water until shells open. While mussels are steaming, sauté garlic in olive oil. Add dill, lemon juice, and wine. Simmer for three minutes. When mussels are open, put on serving plate and pour mixture over each. Serves two.

Salmon Steaks in Curry Sauce

Two 8-ounce salmon steaks
2 tsp curry powder
1 tsp turmeric

½ tsp cayenne pepper
1 c chicken stock (salt free)
4 tsp white wine

Wash salmon, and place in shallow baking dish. Mix curry, turmeric, and pepper with chicken stock, and pour over fish. Pour in white wine, and cover with foil. Bake at 350 degrees for twenty to thirty minutes. Salmon should flake easily with fork. Serves two.

Chez Lorraine's Baked Salmon

4 salmon steaks (about 1¾–2 lb)
4 T lemon juice
1 tsp dill weed

2 T finely chopped fresh chives
Lime wedges

Place each salmon steak on a piece of aluminum foil large enough to wrap it. Pour lemon juice over each steak, sprinkle with dill, and seal each steak in its aluminum pouch. Put the aluminum-sealed steaks in a Pyrex dish and bake at 350 degrees for thirty minutes or until the fish flakes easily with a fork. Serve salmon with sprinkled chives and lime wedges. Serves four.

Shrimp-Stuffed Avocados

4 large avocados, peeled
  and halved, seeds removed
1½ c small salad shrimp,
  cooked and washed

1 T lemon juice
1 T onion powder
1 tsp black pepper
1 T paprika

Set avocados on serving plate with cut side facing up. Combine shrimp, lemon juice, onion powder, and pepper in a medium-size mixing bowl. Spoon shrimp mixture onto each avocado, covering generously. Sprinkle top of each stuffed avocado with paprika before serving. Serves four.

Barbecued Alaskan Shrimp

2½ lb shelled and steamed
  jumbo shrimp with tails
  left on
¼ c virgin olive oil
3 garlic cloves, minced

⅛ tsp paprika
Dash of cayenne pepper
2 T lemon juice
2 fresh limes, cut into wedges
3–4 sprigs fresh parsley

Place cooked shrimp in a large bowl. Mix olive oil, garlic, spices, and lemon juice in a separate bowl. Brush shrimp with spice mixture, and place on hot grill or under broiler for one to two minutes. Turn shrimp and continue cooking for an additional one to two minutes. Garnish with lime wedges and parsley. Serves three to four.

Tahoe Shrimp Salad

1 lb small salad shrimp,
  cooked
½ red onion, minced
1 T dried dill weed
1 T paprika

2 T fresh-squeezed lemon
  juice
3 c chopped lettuce
1 hard-boiled egg, sliced

Rinse and drain shrimp, and set aside. In a small bowl, mix together onion, dill weed, paprika, and lemon juice. Fold in shrimp. Serve shrimp salad on lettuce, and top with hard-boiled egg slices. Serves two.

Red Snapper in Snappy Sauce

¼ c olive oil
2 cloves garlic
2 lb red snapper filets
½ c freshly squeezed lime juice
2 T freshly squeezed lemon
  juice
1 tsp cayenne pepper

1 tsp black pepper
2 tomatoes, diced
4 scallions, sliced thin
½ green bell pepper, chopped
½ red bell pepper, chopped
Cilantro for garnish

Heat oil in skillet, and sauté garlic until golden brown. Lay fish in oil, and sprinkle with lime and lemon juice. Sprinkle cayenne and black peppers over all, then add tomatoes, scallions, and red and green bell peppers. Cover and simmer for fifteen minutes or until fish flakes easily with a fork. Garnish with cilantro. Serves four.

Brockway Tuna Salad

1 can albacore tuna, packed
  in water, low sodium
½ red onion, chopped
½ c chopped celery
1 small jar diced pimentos
  (no salt)

½ c Omega 3 Mayonnaise
1 c shredded romaine lettuce
1 T flaxseed oil
1 T lemon juice
1 tsp paprika
½ tsp freshly ground pepper

Drain tuna, then place in a colander and rinse thoroughly to remove any remaining salt. In a mixing bowl, combine tuna with onion, celery, pimentos, and mayonnaise, mixing thoroughly. Toss the lettuce with flaxseed oil and lemon juice, and make a bed of lettuce in a medium-size serving bowl. Dollop the tuna mixture on the lettuce bed. Sprinkle with paprika and pepper to taste. Serves one.

DOMESTIC LOW-FAT MEAT ENTRÉES
(Beef, Chicken, Veal, Pork, Organ Meats, Game Meats)

Beef

Stir-Fried Beef with Vegetables

12 oz boneless sirloin steak, trimmed of all visible fat, thinly sliced into small, bite-size strips
2 T olive oil
1 clove garlic, pressed
¼ c Burgundy wine
1 yellow onion, cut thinly into wedges

1 red pepper, seeded and cut into slender strips
2 celery stalks, chopped
4 oz thinly sliced carrots
4 oz sliced mushrooms
3 T lemon juice

Sauté the beef in half of the oil with garlic and half of the wine until the beef is browned. Remove from skillet. Heat the residual oil in the skillet. Sauté the onion, red pepper, celery, and carrots until the onion is tender—about four minutes. Add the remainder of the wine. Add the mushrooms and lemon juice. Stir-fry mixture for approximately three more minutes. Combine the vegetables with the meat. Serves two.

Omega Meatballs

1 lb lean ground beef
1 T olive oil
1 medium carrot, grated
1 small scallion, finely diced

1 omega 3–enriched egg, beaten
¼ tsp powdered garlic
¼ tsp powdered onion

Mix all ingredients and make into small balls. Place the meatballs in a Pyrex pan greased with olive oil. Bake covered at 350 degrees for thirty to forty-five minutes or until done. Serves two to three.

Beef and Spinach Scramble

2 T olive oil
1 lb very lean ground beef
3 scallions, chopped
2 cloves garlic, minced
1 tsp black pepper

1 tsp basil
1 c fresh spinach, washed and
  steamed
4 omega 3–enriched eggs,
  scrambled

In a large, heavy skillet heat olive oil. Add beef, scallions, garlic, pepper, and basil. Cook on low heat until meat is thoroughly browned. Turn heat up to medium and add spinach, stirring for five minutes. Add eggs and continue stirring for about one minute or until eggs are cooked. Serves four.

Auroch Beef Cabbage Rolls

1 head cabbage
1½ lb very lean ground beef
1 medium red onion, chopped
2 omega 3–enriched eggs
¼ tsp black pepper

1 tsp oregano
1 clove garlic, minced
6–8 medium-size tomatoes,
  peeled and pureed

Wash cabbage and remove core. Steam for five minutes or until leaves are loose and slightly limp. Pull off leaves and set aside. Mix together all remaining ingredients, reserving ⅓ c tomato puree for later. Fill each cabbage leaf with meat mixture and roll. Place in 9 × 13-inch glass baking dish. Spread rolls with remaining tomato puree, and cover with foil. Bake at 350 degrees for one hour. Serves four to six.

Paleo-Correct Meat Loaf

2 lb extra-lean ground beef
2 red onions, finely chopped
4 garlic cloves, minced
½ red pepper, chopped
½ c fresh cilantro, chopped

½ c fresh parsley, chopped
2 tsp cumin
1 tsp pepper
3 omega 3–enriched eggs, beaten
2 T olive oil

Mix all ingredients in a large mixing bowl. Spread mixture evenly in an 8½ × 11-inch baking dish. Bake at 400 degrees for forty-five minutes or until well cooked. Serves eight.

Burgundy Walnut Beef Roast

1 beef roast (2–3 lb)
6 large tomatoes, diced
¼ tsp black pepper
2 garlic cloves, minced
1 c Burgundy wine

1 red onion, diced
2 T freshly squeezed lemon juice
3 T olive oil
1 T dry mustard

Place meat in covered deep roasting pan. Mix all other ingredients, and pour over meat. Cover and bake at 350 degrees for one to one and a half hours, and baste two or three times while baking. Serves six.

Chicken

Kenny's Barbecued Spicy Chicken

2 T fresh lemon juice
1 T fresh orange juice
2 scallions, finely chopped
1 tsp finely chopped fresh
  tarragon
1 tsp finely chopped fresh thyme
1 tsp finely chopped fresh sage

1 tsp fennel seeds, toasted
  and crushed
Freshly ground black pepper
  to taste
4 boneless, skinless chicken
  breast halves

In a large bowl combine all ingredients except chicken. Mix well to produce marinade. Place the chicken in the bowl, coat thoroughly, and marinate for one to two hours. For grilling: Fire up the barbecue and grill the chicken on medium heat, turning constantly while basting with the marinade until the breasts are cooked. For broiling: Cook under the broiler, turning constantly while basting with the marinade until done. Serves four.

Altamira Stuffed Chicken

½ red onion, chopped
1 T olive oil
3–4 chopped chicken livers
½ c Pinot Noir red wine
¼ c raisins

½ c walnuts
¼ c celery
1 apple, cored, peeled,
  and diced
1 whole, skinned large chicken

Sauté onion in oil until tender. Mix in chopped chicken livers and brown. Pour in wine, add raisins, walnuts, celery, and apple, and simmer for five minutes. Stuff chicken with mixture and bake in covered dish at 400 degrees for one hour or until done. Serves three to four.

Gingery Chicken and Veggies

½ c olive oil
2 cloves garlic, minced
½ red onion, sliced
1 tsp powdered ginger
2 c cooked chicken breast
    meat, skinless and diced

1 c chicken broth
    (no salt)
½ c chopped celery
1 c thinly sliced carrots
½ bell pepper, sliced

Heat oil mixture in heavy skillet, and sauté garlic and onion. Add remaining ingredients and simmer until vegetables are tender. Serves four.

Chicken Cacciatore

2 whole skinned chickens,
    cut up and trimmed
    of visible fat
1 tsp pepper
1 tsp oregano
1 red onion, sliced
1 c sliced mushrooms

4 celery stalks, cut in
    ½ inch pieces
½ c water
8 tomatoes, diced
1 tsp basil
1 tsp parsley

Place chicken pieces in large baking dish. Sprinkle with pepper and oregano. Lay onion, mushrooms, and celery on top of chicken pieces. Pour in ½ c water to cover bottom of dish. Spread tomatoes over chicken, and top with sprinkles of basil and parsley. Bake at 325 degrees for two hours or until chicken is done. Serves six.

Veal

Slow-Cooked Veal with Salsa

2 lb veal, sliced ½ inch thick
2 c tomato salsa (recipe below)

Place veal slices in crock pot, cover with salsa, and cook on low heat for five hours. Remove from pot and pour remaining salsa over meat before serving. Serves four.

Salsa

6 large tomatoes, diced
1 yellow onion, minced
3 cloves garlic, minced
1 tsp black pepper

½ c lime juice
1 tsp cayenne pepper
⅓ c finely chopped
    fresh cilantro

Combine all ingredients and mix well. Makes 2 cups.

Sicilian Skillet Veal Chops

8 veal chops
4 T olive oil
Pepper to taste
1 T oregano

1 T chopped parsley
2 garlic cloves, minced
2 lb tomatoes skinned, boiled,
    and mashed

In your largest skillet, brown chops in oil. Season with pepper. Sprinkle with oregano and parsley. Add garlic and tomatoes. Cover and simmer until tender, about thirty to forty minutes. Serves eight.

Pork

Pork Chops Stuffed with Chicken Livers

6 double rib lean pork chops,
    trimmed of all visible fat
4 T olive oil
6 chicken livers, chopped

½ lb mushrooms, chopped
Pepper to taste
1 T finely chopped parsley

Slit chops to make pockets. Sauté the livers and mushrooms in 2 T of the olive oil. Season the chops with pepper and add parsley. Stuff pork chips with liver mixture and skewer to close pockets. Heat the remaining oil in a heavy skillet, add chops, and sear them over high heat on both sides. Place in large casserole dish, and bake at 350 degrees for twenty-five minutes or until tender. Serves six.

Broiled Tenderloin of Pork with Spicy Rub

1 garlic clove, minced
1 T paprika
1 T dry mustard
1 T ground coriander
2 T olive oil

1 T red wine
1 lb very lean pork tenderloin,
   trimmed of all visible fat
   and cut butterflied down
   the middle

Mix garlic and dry spices in a mortar and pestle. Add in the oil and wine to make a paste. Rub the paste on the butterflied pork one hour before broiling. Broil pork 2 to 3 inches from heat source for about six minutes per side or until it is cooked to desired condition. Serves four.

Isola Baked Pork Chops

4 tomatoes, quartered
1½ c peeled and diced eggplant
2 c sliced zucchini
½ lb mushrooms, halved
1 clove garlic, minced
1 bay leaf

¼ tsp thyme
¼ tsp basil
¼ tsp chopped parsley
½ tsp black pepper
1 T olive oil
4 lean pork chops

Combine all ingredients except oil and pork chops. Grease a 9 × 13-inch baking dish with oil. Then layer the vegetable and spice mixture on bottom, and place pork chops on top. Cover and bake at 350 degrees for one hour or until meat is tender. Serve the vegetables as a separate dish. Serves four.

ORGAN MEATS

Lorrie's Liver and Onions

¼ c olive oil
1 red onion, sliced thin
2 cloves garlic, minced
½ tsp basil

½ tsp rosemary
1 lb calf's liver
½ c Burgundy wine

Heat oil in heavy skillet. Sauté onion, garlic, basil, and rosemary until onions are tender. Add liver, reduce heat, and simmer for ten minutes. Pour in wine and continue to simmer for fifteen minutes. Serves four.

Sautéed Rocky Mountain Chicken Livers

1 medium yellow onion, diced
2 garlic cloves, minced
1 green pepper, diced

2 T olive oil
¼ c Burgundy wine
1 lb chicken livers

Sauté the onion, garlic, and pepper in the oil with half of the wine. Add the livers and remaining wine. Sauté the livers until they are firm and brown. Serves four.

GAME MEATS

Buffalo Burgers

1 lb ground buffalo
½ red onion, finely chopped
2 garlic cloves, minced

1 T basil
1 T oregano
2 tsp black pepper

Mix all ingredients together in large mixing bowl until well blended. Shape meat into patties, and grill or broil on low heat, turning often. Serves four.

Tender Buffalo Roast

3–4 lb buffalo roast
1 red onion, chopped
1 small turnip, chopped
2 carrots, sliced thin
2 cloves garlic, minced

½ tsp black pepper
1 c red wine
⅓ c water
3 T chopped parsley

Place meat in a large baking dish. Add all remaining ingredients. Cover and cook at 400 degrees for ninety minutes or until meat is done through to the center. Slice thinly and place on serving plate. Pour remaining juices over meat before serving. Serves six.

Rocky Mountain Elk Steaks

4 medium-size elk steaks   1 tsp ground sage
½ c olive oil   1 tsp basil
2 garlic cloves, minced   1 tsp rosemary
½ red onion, sliced   1 c Burgundy wine

Wash steaks thoroughly, and place in 9 × 13-inch baking dish. Heat olive oil on low heat in heavy skillet. Sauté garlic, onion, and spices until tender. Stir in wine, and remove from heat. Pour over elk steaks. Cover and refrigerate for two to three hours. Grill or broil slowly until cooked as desired. Serves four.

Roast Pheasant with Fruit and Nut Stuffing

1 pheasant (2–3 lb)   3 cloves
¼ c olive oil   ½ tsp ginger
1 T fresh ground pepper   ½ c dried and coarsely chopped
1 T garlic powder   apricots (nonsulfured)
1½ c freshly squeezed orange   ½ tsp grated orange peel
  juice   1 c chopped pecans
½ c raisins

Preheat oven to 350 degrees. Wash and dry the pheasant, and brush with olive oil inside and out. Sprinkle inside and out with pepper and garlic powder. In a saucepan, combine the orange juice, raisins, and cloves. Bring to a boil, reduce the heat, and simmer for five minutes. Strain the mixture, discarding the cloves and reserving the orange juice and raisins. In a mixing bowl, combine the orange juice/raisin mixture, ginger, apricots, orange peel, and nuts. Mix well and use to stuff the pheasant. Place the pheasant, breast up, on a rack in a roasting pan and roast until tender, about thirty minutes per pound; brush frequently with the remaining orange juice. Place the pheasant on a serving platter, and trickle the liquid from the roasting pan over the pheasant. Serves two.

Barbecued Venison Steaks with Herbs

2 T chopped rosemary   ¼ c olive oil
2 T chopped garlic   4 venison steaks (4 oz each)
2 T chopped thyme   Fresh ground pepper to taste

Make a marinade by combining the herbs and olive oil in a mixing bowl. Marinate the venison for four hours in refrigerator, covered. Remove steaks from marinade, and shake off excess oil. For grilling: Place steaks on grill, season with pepper, and brush frequently with marinade. Cook the steaks for about two to four minutes per side until well cooked. For broiling: Place steaks on broiler in oven for about five minutes per side or until cooked to your taste. Serves four.

DRIED MEATS (JERKY)

Basic Beef Jerky

2 lb lean beef, trimmed of all visible fat, cut into 1-inch-wide,
⅛-inch-thick strips with the grain of the muscle when possible

The easiest way to make jerky is to buy your own food dryer. Place beef strips on the racks of a home food dryer (available at any large discount store), and dry the meat until it is tough and chewy (usually overnight). Alternatively, dry in your oven on ungreased cookie sheets. Set oven at lowest baking temperature, and keep the door propped open. Maintain the temperature between 140 and 150 degrees. Drying time varies among ovens but typically takes from four to twelve hours. The jerky is done when it is chewy and tough.

Spicy Beef Jerky

2 lb lean beef, trimmed of all visible fat, cut into 1-inch-wide,
⅛-inch-thick strips. (Almost any meat can be dried; try lean pork, venison, buffalo, even poultry and fish.) Follow instructions above for drying.

Chili powder	Lemon pepper
Cumin	Turmeric
Garlic powder	Coarse ground black pepper
Onion powder	Curry powder
Dry mustard	White pepper
Cayenne pepper	

Mix any and all combinations of the spices listed above in a medium-size bowl to make a dry rub. Let your personal taste and imagination guide you, varying the amount of each ingredient according to preference. Our favorite is equal amounts of cumin, garlic powder, coarse ground black pepper, turmeric, and cayenne pepper. Dip each meat strip in the bowl of spices. Lightly coat and then marinate for at least thirty minutes; it's better if you have time to marinate the meat overnight in a covered bowl in the refrigerator. Then prepare jerky using method in recipe above.

Dried Salmon

2 lb salmon filets cut into ½- to 1-inch-wide, ⅛-inch-thick strips.
   Include the skin and try to use wild, rather than farmed,
   salmon. Wild salmon tastes much better.

Dry the salmon strips using the same method as with the beef jerky. Again, the easiest way is to use your own food dryer. Place the salmon strips on the racks of a home food dryer (available at any large discount store), and dry the meat until it is not hard but just a little chewy. The oven-baking method also works.

EGG DISHES
Zesty Shrimp-Avocado Omelet

2 omega 3–enriched eggs
1 T olive oil
1 T chopped scallions
1 T chopped tomatoes
¼ c small shrimp
   (fresh or thawed frozen)

1 tsp dried dill weed
½ tsp black pepper
Guacamole Fiesta
   (see page 189 for recipe)

Crack eggs into a small bowl, and mix thoroughly with a fork or a wire whisk. Using a small, nonstick omelet skillet, heat oil on medium heat. Pour in eggs, and cook slowly until bubbles appear in the middle. Using a spatula, gently lift edges of omelet and allow uncooked egg to run off to sides. Once the omelet is firm, sprinkle scallions, tomatoes, and shrimp in center of omelet, and top with dill and pepper. Fold omelets in half, and cook for 30 seconds. Remove from pan, and top with Guacamole Fiesta. Serves one.

Scrambled Basil Eggs Topped
with Salsa

2 omega 3–enriched eggs
1 tsp dried basil

2 T Anaheim Cilantro Salsa
(see page 190 for recipe)

Crack eggs into a small bowl, add basil, and mix thoroughly with a fork or a wire whisk. Scramble eggs in a nonstick skillet. Remove the eggs with a Teflon spatula, and top with Anaheim Cilantro Salsa. Serves one.

Poached Eggs with
Peach Salsa

Olive oil
2 omega 3–enriched eggs

2 T Peach Salsa
(see page 190 for recipe)

Bring ½ inch of water to a boil in a saucepan. Rub a little olive oil in the egg wells of an egg poacher (available at most kitchen and cooking specialty stores). Crack eggs into the egg wells and reduce heat to a slow boil. Place poacher in the saucepan and cover. Extra-large eggs take about seven minutes for soft yolks; medium eggs, about six minutes. Remove egg poacher from pan with a hot glove, and free the eggs with a flexible rubber spatula. Gently transfer the eggs to a plate, and smother with Peach Salsa. Serves one.

VEGETABLE DISHES
Carrot-Mushroom Stir-Fry

6 carrots, sliced thin
4 T olive oil
5 scallions, sliced into
   1-inch pieces

10 medium mushrooms,
   sliced thin
1 T lemon juice
½ tsp black pepper

Steam carrots until tender. Heat oil in large skillet. Add carrots, scallions, and mushrooms, and stir-fry until all are cooked. Add lemon juice and pepper, and mix well. Serves four.

Baked Mushrooms Contra Costa

12 large white mushrooms	1 clove garlic, minced
4 T lemon juice	2 T minced onion
2 T olive oil	1 tsp black pepper
2 T minced parsley	2–4 T dry sherry

Wash mushrooms and remove stems. Sprinkle lemon juice on each cap, and set in 9 × 13-inch baking dish. Mince stems and sauté in olive oil. In a medium-size bowl, combine sautéed mushroom stems with remaining ingredients. Spoon stuffing generously into each mushroom cap. Cover and bake at 350 degrees for fifteen minutes. Serves three to four.

Marinated Mushrooms

20 medium mushrooms	¼ c lemon juice
2 red onions, sliced	1 clove garlic, minced
¼ c fresh chopped parsley	¼ tsp black pepper
1 c olive oil	1 tsp oregano
½ c dry white wine	

Wash mushrooms, and slice in half. Combine with onions. In blender, puree remaining ingredients. Pour over mushrooms and onions, mixing well. Refrigerate overnight or longer. Serves four.

Ratatouille

2 large onions, chopped	1 lb diced eggplant
2 cloves garlic, minced	4 large tomatoes, skinned
4 T olive oil	and wedged
2 green peppers, seeded	3 T fresh chopped parsley
and cut into strips	½ tsp oregano
1 lb sliced zucchini	¼ tsp black pepper

Sauté onions and garlic in olive oil until tender. Add remaining ingredients, and bring to a boil. Reduce heat, cover, and let simmer until vegetables are tender (about thirty to forty-five minutes). Serves six to eight.

Spicy Stuffed Squash

2 medium acorn squash
½ c water
2 medium carrots, cooked
　　and chopped
2 small turnips, cooked and
　　chopped

1 T olive oil
½ tsp ground cinnamon
¼ tsp nutmeg
1 c peeled, coarsely chopped
　　apple

Cut squash in half, and remove seeds and strings. Place squash, cut side down, in a 9 × 13-inch baking dish. Add water, and cover with foil. Bake at 350 degrees for thirty minutes. Remove from oven, and turn squash so that cut side is facing up. Cover with foil, and bake for twenty to thirty minutes more until tender. Scoop the pulp out of each squash half, keeping shells intact. Place pulp in blender, and add carrots and turnips. Blend until smooth. Stir in oil, cinnamon, and nutmeg, blending well. Fold in apple, and spoon into squash shells. Return to baking dish, and bake at 350 degrees for fifteen to twenty minutes or until heated through. Serves four.

Baked Tomatoes

2 large tomatoes
½ c minced mushrooms
1 tsp chopped parsley
1 clove garlic, minced
1 scallion, chopped

1 tsp finely chopped fresh
　　basil
½ tsp thyme
¼ c olive oil

Slice tomatoes in half, scoop out most of the pulp, and set in medium-size baking dish. Combine pulp with remaining ingredients, and fill each tomato half. Bake at 375 degrees for ten to fifteen minutes. Serves four.

Walnut Broccoli with Carrots

½ c olive oil
1 medium onion, sliced in rings
2 large carrots, sliced
　　diagonally ⅛ inch thick

2 large stalks broccoli, sliced
　　¼ inch thick
½ c raw, shelled walnuts

Heat oil in heavy skillet, and sauté onion until tender. Add carrots and broccoli, and stir-fry until tender yet crispy. Add walnuts, and cook three to five minutes longer. Serves two.

SALADS
Spinach Salad à la Cordani

½ lb pork tenderloin, sliced
  and chopped into fine pieces
2 T olive oil
1 bunch fresh spinach, washed,
  drained, and torn into pieces
  of desired size

1 can sliced water chestnuts
  (rinsed of salt)
1 lb fresh mushrooms,
  sliced thin
4 hard-boiled omega 3–
  enriched eggs, sliced

Sauté the pork tenderloin pieces in the olive oil until lightly browned. In a large serving bowl, toss together spinach, water chestnuts, and mushrooms. Top the salad with sliced, hard-boiled eggs and pork tenderloin pieces. Allow diners to add their own favorite dressing (see pages 190–191 for dressing recipes). Serves four.

Ambrosia Salad

6 carrots, shredded
2 c fresh pineapple chunks
¼ c raisins

¼ c walnuts
1 T lemon juice

In large bowl, mix all ingredients. Cover and chill before serving. Serves four.

Spinach Salad with Crabmeat

2 large bunches fresh spinach
  leaves, washed and dried
1 Walla Walla, Vidalia, or Maui
  sweet onion, sliced thin
2 large tomatoes, sliced thin

½ lb cooked, shredded
  crabmeat
2 hard-boiled omega 3–
  enriched eggs, sliced thin

Tear spinach leaves into small pieces, and mix with onions, tomatoes, and crabmeat. Just before serving, toss with Spinach Salad Dressing (see page 190) and top with egg slices. Serves four.

Carrot Salad

8 carrots

1 medium red onion, sliced thin

1 green pepper, seeded and
sliced thin

4 medium tomatoes,
peeled and pureed

½ c flaxseed oil

¾ c lemon juice

4 T dry mustard

½ tsp black pepper

Steam carrots until tender. Slice them thinly crosswise, and place in a large bowl. Combine remaining ingredients until well mixed, and then add to carrots, stirring until carrots are well coated. Refrigerate overnight, and serve well chilled. Serves four.

Almond Chicken Salad

1 c cooked, diced chicken
breast meat

1 c chopped romaine lettuce

1 c shredded butter leaf lettuce

¼ c chopped red cabbage

½ c sliced almonds

¼ c chopped Medjool dates

1–2 T flaxseed oil

1–2 T freshly squeezed orange
juice

Combine all ingredients except liquids in a large serving bowl. Toss with flaxseed oil and freshly squeezed orange juice. Serves two.

Marinated Cauliflower Salad

1 head cauliflower, small florets

½ red onion, sliced

½ green bell pepper, chopped

⅔ c marinade (below)

In medium-size salad bowl, combine cauliflower, onion, and pepper. Pour marinade over entire mixture, and refrigerate overnight. Serves four.

Marinade:

1 tsp black pepper

1 tsp dry mustard

6 tsp lemon juice

3 tsp red wine

1 c flaxseed oil

1 T dried onion flakes

1 T finely chopped fresh
parsley,

Mix all dressing ingredients in blender. Makes 1½ cups.

Butter Leaf Avocado Salad

2 c shredded butter leaf lettuce
1 c chopped iceberg lettuce
¼ c raisins
1 c quartered tomatoes

1 c avocado slices
Avocado oil
Lemon juice

Combine the lettuce, raisins, and tomatoes in a serving bowl, and layer the avocado slices around the top. Dress with avocado oil and lemon juice. Serves three.

Waldorf Salad

2 c diced, unpeeled red apples
2 T lemon juice mixed with
  2 T flaxseed oil
1 c thinly sliced celery

½ c chopped walnuts
½ c raisins
2 c chopped iceberg lettuce
  leaves

Toss together first five ingredients. Serve on top of lettuce bed. Serves two.

CONDIMENTS, DIPS, SALSAS, SALAD DRESSINGS, MARINADES

Omega 3 Mayonnaise

1 whole egg
1 T lemon juice
¼ tsp dry mustard

½ c olive oil
½ c flaxseed oil

Put egg, lemon juice, and mustard in blender, and blend for three to five seconds. Continue blending, and slowly add oils. Blend until the mayonnaise is thick. Scrape mayonnaise into a snaplock plastic container and refrigerate. The mayonnaise should keep for five to seven days. Makes 1 cup.

Veggie Dip

1 c Omega 3 Mayonnaise (recipe above)
1 tsp dried dill

½ tsp garlic powder
Pepper to taste

Mix all ingredients together. It is better if refrigerated for one hour before serving, but it is not necessary. Makes a great dip for raw veggies or to use as a salad dressing. Makes 1 cup.

Tartar Sauce

1 c Omega 3 Mayonnaise
  (recipe above)
¼ c finely chopped red onion
½ T lemon juice

½ tsp dried dill
¼ tsp paprika
Pinch of garlic powder

Mix ingredients together. Chill prior to serving. Makes 1¼ cups.

Ray's Catsup

3½ lb tomatoes, washed
  and sliced
2 medium onions, sliced
⅛ clove garlic
½ bay leaf
½ red pepper
¼ c unsweetened fruit juice
  (white grape, pear, or apple)

1 tsp whole allspice
1 tsp whole cloves
1 tsp whole mace
1 tsp celery seeds
1 tsp black peppercorns
½ inch cinnamon stick
½ c lemon juice
Pinch of cayenne pepper

Boil tomatoes, onions, garlic, bay leaf, and pepper until soft. Add fruit juice. Mix spices (allspice, cloves, mace, celery seeds, peppercorns, and cinnamon), and put into a small cloth spice bag. Add spice bag to mixture; bring to a boil and continue boiling, stirring frequently, until reduced by half. Remove the spice bag. Add lemon juice and cayenne pepper. Continue boiling for ten minutes more. Bottle catsup in clean jars, with ¾ inch of space at top of jar for expansion. Seal and freeze immediately. Always refrigerate container that is currently in use. Makes about 2 cups.

Source: *Neanderthin: A Caveman's Guide to Nutrition,* by Ray Audette. New York: St. Martin's Press, 1999.

Guacamole Fiesta

3 ripe avocados
1 tsp freshly squeezed lemon juice
1 tsp coarsely ground black pepper
1 tsp garlic powder

1 jalapeño pepper, finely
  diced, destemmed, and
  deseeded

Mash avocados together with a fork or potato masher until smooth, and then stir in all other ingredients until well mixed. Makes 1½ cups.

Anaheim Cilantro Salsa

2 garlic cloves
1 large yellow onion, quartered
1 Anaheim pepper,
   quartered and seeded
3 jalapeño peppers

6 tomatoes, peeled,
   seeded, and chopped
1 c fresh cilantro
1 tsp ground cumin
Freshly ground pepper to taste

Mince garlic, onions, and peppers in a blender. Add tomatoes and cilantro, and continue blending until ingredients are mixed but still slightly chunky. Add cumin and pepper. Refrigerate until ready to use. Makes 2 cups.

Peach Salsa

1 c fresh peaches, peeled
   and finely chopped
¼ c chopped red onions
¼ c chopped yellow or green
   peppers

1 T lime juice
2 tsp chopped fresh cilantro
Cayenne pepper to taste

In a medium-size bowl, stir all ingredients together. Cover and chill for up to 6 hours. Makes 2 cups.

Spinach Salad Dressing

3 T dry mustard
1 clove garlic, minced
1 T black pepper
1 tsp cayenne pepper
1 tsp paprika

1 c Burgundy wine
1 c fresh tomatoes, pureed
2 c flaxseed oil
1 c lemon juice

Combine all ingredients in blender. Pour into a cruet, and shake well before each use. Makes 5 cups.

Omega 3 Russian Salad Dressing

1 c fresh tomatoes
½ c flaxseed oil
½ c lemon juice
3 T freshly squeezed orange juice
1 tsp paprika

1 small scallion or
   1 tsp onion powder
1 tsp horseradish powder
   (optional)
1 garlic clove (optional)

Put all ingredients in a blender, and blend until smooth. Makes 1 cup.

Raspberry Barbecue Sauce

2 tsp olive oil
¼ c minced onion
1 T seeded and minced
  jalapeño chili
¼ c Ray's Catsup (see page
  189 for recipe)

¼ tsp dry mustard
¼ tsp cayenne pepper
2 c fresh or frozen
  raspberries

Heat oil in a heavy skillet, and sauté onion and chili for about ten minutes. Add catsup, mustard, and cayenne, and heat until simmering. Add raspberries, and simmer for an additional ten minutes. Remove from heat and let cool. Pour into blender, and blend until smooth. Makes about 1½ cups.

Kona Local Marinade

½ c unsweetened fresh
  pineapple juice
¼ c olive oil

3 T lime juice
2 T finely grated fresh
  gingerroot

Combine all ingredients in a small bowl, and whisk until well blended. Use to marinate beef, chicken, pork, or fish when barbecuing. Makes about 1 cup.

Garlic and Herb Marinade

4 cloves garlic
4 T olive oil
⅓ c chopped fresh basil
⅓ c chopped fresh oregano

⅓ c chopped fresh parsley
6 T lemon juice
1 tsp black pepper

Mince garlic, and place in blender. Add remaining ingredients, and blend until well mixed. Use to brush on vegetables, chicken, or meat before and during grilling or broiling. Makes one-half cup.

SOUPS

Chicken Vegetable Soup

6 c water
Meat of 1 whole chicken,
  diced
2 cloves garlic, minced
1 yellow onion, diced

1 bay leaf
1 tsp black pepper
6 fresh tomatoes, diced
2 small zucchini, sliced thin
3 carrots, diced

In a large pot, combine water, chicken, garlic, onion, bay leaf, and pepper. Bring to a boil. Reduce heat, cover, and simmer for about two hours or until chicken is tender. Remove bay leaf and discard. Add remaining ingredients, and bring to a boil. Reduce heat and cover. Simmer for about twenty minutes or until vegetables are tender. Serves six.

Gazpacho

4 large tomatoes, chopped
1 small onion, coarsely chopped
1 clove garlic, peeled
1 c unsalted tomato juice
2 T lemon juice
Pepper to taste

Cayenne pepper to taste
  (optional)
1 sprig fresh parsley
4 ice cubes
1 medium cucumber, peeled
  and coarsely chopped

Blend all ingredients in a blender or food processor until vegetables are small but not pureed. Serves two.

Source: Cooking Healthy with One Foot Out the Door by Polly Pritchford and Delia Quigley. Summertown, TN: The Book Publishing Company, 1995.

Paleo Zucchini Soup

2 T olive oil
1 red onion, chopped
5 cloves garlic, minced
2 qts water
2 c cooked, chopped beef,
  chicken, or pork
2 T dried basil
2 T dried parsley

2 T dried thyme
1 T black pepper
2 c chopped carrots
2 c chopped celery
2 c chopped zucchini
2 c fresh chopped
  tomatoes
½ c fresh chopped parsley

Heat olive oil, and sauté onion and garlic. Bring water to a boil, and add sautéed onion and garlic, meat, basil, parsley, thyme, and pepper. Lower heat, and simmer for one hour. One hour before eating, add carrots and celery. One-half hour before eating, add zucchini. Ten minutes before eating, add chopped tomatoes and fresh parsley. Serves six.

Spicy Tomato Soup

8 fresh tomatoes, pureed
1 c water
¼ c diced green chilies
1 c chicken broth
1 red onion, finely minced

2 cloves garlic, minced
¼ c diced chives
1 bell pepper, diced
1 tsp cayenne pepper
1 tsp paprika

Combine all ingredients in a large soup pot, and cook on low heat for one hour. Serves six.

FRUIT DISHES AND DESSERTS

Kyle's Apple Breakfast

1 large apple (any type),
    chopped into bite-size pieces
1 medium carrot, grated

Handful of raisins
Cinnamon

Mix the apple, carrot, and raisins in a bowl, and sprinkle cinnamon over the top. Serves one.

Almost Frozen Mashed Bananas

3–4 ripe bananas
1 tsp natural vanilla extract

Mash bananas with fork or potato masher in a bowl, and thoroughly stir in vanilla. Put mixture in freezer for twenty to thirty minutes, until it is thick but not frozen solid. Serves three to four.

Fresh Cinnamon Applesauce

6 apples   1 tsp cinnamon
2–3 T fresh lemon juice

Core, peel, and slice apples. Combine with lemon juice in blender
until smooth. Sprinkle with cinnamon and serve. Serves two.

Emerald Bay Fruit and Nut Mix

½ c walnuts   ½ c almonds
½ c pecans   ½ c chopped Medjool dates
½ c raisins   2 T lemon juice
½ c chopped fresh apples   1 tsp cinnamon

Combine all nuts and fruits in a large serving bowl. Mix in lemon
juice and cinnamon. Serve in small bowls. Serves four.

Baked Walnut-Cinnamon Apples

4 apples   ¼ tsp cinnamon
1 c raisins   ½ tsp natural vanilla extract
¼ c chopped walnuts   ½ c water

Heat oven to 375 degrees. Core and pierce apples with a fork in
several places around the center, to prevent them from bursting.
Mix raisins, nuts, cinnamon, and vanilla in a small bowl. Fill center
of each apple with this mixture. Place in a glass baking dish, and
pour water into pan. Cover with foil, and bake for about thirty
minutes or until tender. Serves four.

Peach-Almond Delight

3 fresh peaches   1 tsp natural vanilla extract
4 oz slivered almonds   2 tsp cinnamon
2 T diced Medjool dates

Wash the peaches, and cut each one into eight sections. Mix with
the almonds and dates, and drizzle with vanilla; sprinkle cinnamon
on top. Serves two.

Cantaloupe Stuffed with Blackberries
and Pecans

1 cantaloupe
1 c blackberries
½ c chopped pecans

Mint or spearmint leaves
for garnish

Cut cantaloupe in half (using a serrated knife), and scoop out seeds. Fill each cavity with blackberries and pecans. Garnish with mint or spearmint leaves. Serves two.

Strawberry-Blueberry Horizon

1 c fresh strawberries
1 c fresh blueberries
½ tangerine, sectioned
1 T freshly squeezed orange juice

1 tsp natural vanilla extract
Ground nutmeg
Fresh mint

Mix the strawberries, blueberries, and tangerine sections in a bowl. Drip with orange juice and vanilla, and sprinkle with nutmeg. Serve chilled and garnished with mint. Serves three.

11

Paleo Exercise

Eating alone will not keep a man well; he must also take exercise.

—Hippocrates

Regular physical activity is every bit as important as diet in achieving good health and permanent weight loss. Regular exercise can:

- Improve your insulin metabolism
- Increase HDL cholesterol and reduce blood triglycerides
- Lower your blood pressure
- Strengthen your heart and blood vessels
- Reduce your risk of developing heart disease and type 2 diabetes
- Alleviate stress, improve your mental outlook, and help you to sleep better
- Possibly increase bone mineral density in people under thirty and slow bone loss in older people

Here again, we need to follow the example set by our hunter-gatherer ancestors and use their activity levels as a guide for our own.

I must tell you that when asked to choose between doing long, hard, repetitive work and simply relaxing, or having fun, hunter-gatherers—just like their modern descendants—invariably would have opted for the latter two choices. In fact, the idea of exercise itself would have baffled these people. After all, no reasonable hunter-gatherers would have lifted heavy stones or run in circles for the mere sake of getting a "workout." Convincing them to continue these boring activities—or to develop a fitness plan—would have been impossible.

The huge difference between Paleolithic people and us is that they had no choice but to do hard manual labor on a regular basis. Their lives depended on it. Most of ours do not.

Exercise Plus Paleo Diet Equals Health: Joe's Story

Joe Friel is an internationally known expert on fitness who has coached Olympic triathletes and is the author of a number of best-selling books for triathletes and cyclists. Here are his experiences with Paleo diets:

> I have known Dr. Cordain for many years, but I didn't become aware of his work until 1995. That year we began to discuss nutrition for sports. As a longtime adherent to a very-high-carbohydrate diet for athletes, I was skeptical of his claim that eating less starch would benefit performance. Nearly every successful endurance athlete I had known ate as I did, with a heavy emphasis on cereals, bread, rice, pasta, pancakes, and potatoes. In fact, I had done quite well on this diet, having been an All-American age-group duathlete (bike and run), finishing in the top ten at World Championships. I had also coached many successful athletes, both professional and amateur, who ate the same way I did.
>
> Our discussions eventually led to a challenge. Dr. Cordain suggested I try eating a diet more in line with what he recommended for one month. I took the challenge, determined to show him that eating as I had for years was the way to go. I started by simply cutting back significantly on starches and replacing those lost calories with fruits, vegetables, and very lean meats.
>
> For the first two weeks I felt miserable. My recovery following workouts was slow, and my workouts were sluggish. I knew that I was well on my way to proving that he was wrong. But in week three, a curious thing happened. I began to notice that I was not only feeling better, but that my recovery was speeding up significantly. In the fourth week I experimented to see how many hours I could train.
>
> Since my early forties (I was fifty-one at the time), I had not been able to train more than about twelve hours per week. Whenever I exceeded this weekly volume, upper-respiratory infections

would soon set me back. In week four of the "experiment," I trained sixteen hours without a sign of a cold, a sore throat, or an ear infection. I was amazed. I hadn't done that many hours in nearly ten years. I decided to keep the experiment going.

That year I finished third at the U.S. national championship, with an excellent race, and qualified for the U.S. team for the World Championships. I had a stellar season, one of my best in years. This, of course, led to more questions of Dr. Cordain and my continued refining of the diet he recommended.

I was soon recommending it to the athletes I coached, including Ryan Bolton, who was on the U.S. Olympic Triathlon team. Since 1995 I have written four books on training for endurance athletes and have described and recommended the Paleo Diet in each of them. Many athletes have told me a story similar to mine: they have tried eating this way, somewhat skeptically at first, and then discovered that they also recovered faster and trained better.

"Exercise": A Funny Idea to Hunter-Gatherers

In the late 1980s, the world community became increasingly alarmed at the shrinking tropical rain forest in the Amazon basin (due to clear-cut logging, mining, and industrialization). Politicians and environmentalists launched a host of programs to curb this deforestation and even brought native Amazon Indians to environmental conferences in New York City. At one such conference, a group of Indians came across joggers exercising in Central Park—and found this concept absolutely hilarious. That adults would run for no apparent reason was comically absurd to these practical hunters. In their tropical forest home, every movement had a function and a purpose. What could possibly be gained by running to no destination, with no predators or enemies to escape from, and with nothing to capture?

Physical Fitness: Naturally, and with No Exercise Programs

The mind-set of these Amazonian Indians was undoubtedly very similar to that of any of the world's hunter-gatherers. They got plenty of exercise simply by carrying out the day's basic activities—finding food and water, building shelters, making tools, and gathering wood. These activities were more than enough to allow them to develop superb physical fitness. Strength, stamina, and good muscle tone were the natural by-products of their daily routine.

Our Stone Age ancestors worked hard or they didn't eat. Sustained labor wasn't necessary every day; periods of intense exertion generally alternated with days of rest and relaxation. But the work was always there, an inevitable fact of life. There were no retirement plans, no vacations, and definitely no labor-saving devices. Everybody, except for the very young or the very old, helped out. And their daily efforts were astonishing. The amount of physical activity performed by an average hunter-gatherer would have been about four times greater than that of a sedentary office worker—and about three times greater than anybody needs to get the health benefits of exercise. An office worker who jogged 3 miles a day for a whole week would use less than half the energy of an average hunter-gatherer, such as the !Kung people of Africa. !Kung men on average walk 9.3 miles per day; the women average 5.7 miles per day. As you may expect, all this walking and regular physical activity pays off with high levels of physical fitness for everyone. In fact, my research team has shown that the average aerobic capacity of the world's hunter-gatherers and less Westernized peoples is similar to that of today's top athletes.

Exercise and Obesity

There are few physicians or health professionals who would argue that exercise shouldn't accompany dietary programs.

Most of the scientific experiments that have monitored weight loss with and without exercise programs have shown that moderate exercise (**20** to **60** minutes of walking or jogging five times a week) doesn't help you lose weight any faster—but it is very effective in helping you keep the extra pounds off over the long term

Why Exercise by Itself Doesn't Promote Weight Loss

The idea of exercising the extra pounds away—if this is your only means of weight loss—is not terribly practical. Exercise combined with diet is no more effective than diet alone in causing weight loss. How can this be? The answer is a scientific equation: to lose a pound of fat, you need to achieve a caloric deficit of 3,500 calories.

Imagine that a mildly obese woman, weighing 154 pounds, would like to lose 30 pounds, or 105,000 calories, by walking or jogging for 3 miles (forty-five minutes) a day. On days when she walks or jogs, she expends 215 additional calories (compared to the 80 calories she expends for that same forty-five-minute period on other days). The 3-mile walk/jog causes a net deficit of 135 calories—not a lot, considering the amount of work she's doing. At this rate, it will take her 26 days to lose 1 pound and 780 days (more than 2 years) to lose 30 pounds. Most dieters simply don't have the patience to wait that long. (Frankly, most of us need the encouragement of seeing the scale change more rapidly to help us keep up the good work. Otherwise, it's easy to become discouraged and give up.)

Experiments by my colleague Dr. Joe Donnelly and coworkers at the University of Nebraska at Kearney, and by Dr. David Nieman at Appalachian State University in Boone, North Carolina, have demonstrated that *diet alone is just as effective as diet plus exercise in causing weight loss.*

The real benefit from exercise for weight loss comes not from the modest caloric deficit that it may create, but from its ability to *keep weight off* once it has been lost. Dr. Rena Wing of Brown University School of Medicine in Providence, Rhode Island, reviewed a large number of exercise trials in which participants either dieted only or dieted and exercised. Reporting on the participants a year later, Dr. Wing noted, "In all of the long-term randomized trials reviewed, weight losses at follow-up were greater in *diet plus exercise* than in *diet only.*"

Why Should You Exercise?

Regular exercise, though, is great for your body. One major benefit: it improves your insulin metabolism. As I've discussed earlier in this book, many overweight people are insensitive to insulin, a hormone secreted by the pancreas that aids the entry of glucose from the bloodstream into all cells of the body, including the muscle cells. When muscle cells become insensitive to insulin, the pancreas responds by secreting more insulin. This, in turn, raises the normal level of insulin in the bloodstream. The resulting elevation of blood insulin levels, called "hyperinsulinemia," is the underlying cause of the metabolic syndrome diseases. Insulin is a master hormone that influences many other critical cellular functions. An elevated level of insulin in the bloodstream encourages fat deposition and the development of obesity.

Regular exercise has been shown in clinical studies to improve the muscles' sensitivity to insulin and to lower the level of insulin in the bloodstream. In other words, although exercise alone does not cause the large caloric deficits needed for weight loss, it sets the metabolic stage for weight loss to occur by improving your insulin metabolism—as long as you cut back on calories.

Improving your insulin sensitivity may also reduce your appetite by preventing the large swings in blood sugar levels that are a direct consequence of too much insulin secretion. When you eat a carbohydrate-heavy meal, digestive enzymes convert most of the carbohydrate to glucose, which then enters the bloodstream. Normally, the pancreas secretes just the right amount of insulin to help convert glucose into muscle and other cells of the body and to help keep the blood sugar level on an even keel. However, when your muscles are resistant to insulin's action and the pancreas must secrete extra insulin, this drives the blood glucose level even lower. This reduction in blood sugar, called "hypoglycemia," makes you hungry—even if you've just eaten a large meal. Exercise can help break this vicious cycle by making the muscles more sensitive to insulin.

Exercise and Blood Lipids

Medical evidence suggests that exercise training alone has little or no effect on the LDL blood cholesterol level. However, it can improve the total/HDL cholesterol ratio and reduce your risk of heart disease by significantly increasing the good HDL blood cholesterol level. Also, exercise has been shown to lower the triglyceride level, which may also be an independent risk factor for atherosclerosis and coronary heart disease.

The best way to improve your levels of total and HDL cholesterol is through a combination of exercise and diet. Do your heart a favor when you adopt the Paleo Diet and start to exercise as well.

Exercise Prevents Heart Disease and High Blood Pressure

Exercise can also decrease your risk of dying from heart disease by triggering a variety of other healthful changes in your heart and circulatory system. Regular physical exertion has been shown to widen and increase the elasticity of the coronary arteries that carry blood to the heart. This widening is good: Even if there are plaques, or chunky deposits, in the coronary arteries of people who regularly exercise, their chances of having a heart attack are reduced because these arteries are wider—which makes it less likely that any blockage will completely cut off blood flow to the heart. With regular exercise, the heart gets bigger and stronger and may even develop new blood vessels to supply more blood and oxygen.

Also, exciting new evidence suggests that regular physical exertion may reduce the risk of a blood clot forming in a coronary artery—a key event leading to a heart attack. The net result of all these beneficial changes from physical activity is a significant reduction in your risk of dying from all forms of heart and blood vessel diseases. This has been demonstrated in a medical study of more than 40,000 women from Iowa.

The most pervasive of all chronic Western diseases is hypertension, or high blood pressure. It affects at least 50 million Americans, and by age sixty-five almost 60 percent of all Americans have blood pressure that is too high. Blood pressure is measured when the heart contracts (this is called "systolic pressure") and when it relaxes ("diastolic pressure"). You are considered to have hypertension if your systolic blood pressure readings are 140 or greater and if your diastolic readings are 90 or greater. Many studies have demonstrated that regular exercise alone—without other lifestyle changes—is effective in lowering blood pressure. Because hypertension can accelerate the risk of stroke, exercise programs that lower blood pressure may also reduce the risk of stroke. Exercise, along with the foods you will be eating on the Paleo Diet, will put you on the right track for lowering your blood pressure and reducing your risk of developing the diseases of the heart and the blood vessels.

Exercise, Type 2 Diabetes, and Other Health Benefits of Exercise

Type 2 diabetes affects an estimated 17 million Americans and normally arises from insulin resistance—the same dangerous condition that promotes obesity, hypertension, heart disease, and blood lipid abnormalities. Exercise can be of great help: a single round of exercise improves insulin sensitivity within three hours and keeps working all day long—even twenty-four hours after your exertion.

Exercise is one of nature's best cures for whatever ails you. Regular physical exertion can reduce stress and optimize your mental well-being, help you sleep better, improve your digestion and lung function, reduce bone mineral loss, and slow the physical changes associated with aging. It may decrease your risk of developing certain types of cancer. So go for it! Embrace the active lifestyle that is part of your ancestral heritage. Activity and movement are built into your genes. Your body absolutely requires it.

Modern Exercises for Your Paleolithic Body

Any activity is better than no activity. It doesn't have to be some ambitious plan devised by a personal trainer. Basically, whenever you can exert yourself physically—at work, at home, while traveling, or during leisure time—you should do it. On a typical day, most Americans walk about 30 feet from the house to the car, drive to work, walk 100 feet to the office, and sit virtually motionless in front of a computer for hours at a time. At the end of the day, they walk back to their cars, drive home, and then sit motionless in front of a TV screen until they go to sleep. Even in once highly active professions, such as construction, it is now possible to do almost as little physical activity as somebody performing a desk job. Operating an air-conditioned backhoe with fully hydraulic controls takes barely more effort than operating a personal computer.

Increasing Your Activity Level While at Home or at Work

In this highly mechanized, technological world, you can increase your physical exertion level while doing your daily tasks at home or at work, during your leisure activities, and by incorporating a regular exercise routine into your schedule. I encourage you to take full advantage of all three of these situations to get activity back into your life. At every occasion when you have the chance to use your body, you should. Look upon activity not as something you have to do but rather as a fleeting opportunity to give your body a gift. Get it when you can! You'll feel better when you do.

Is it possible for you to sneak in some exercise on the way to or from work? Could you walk to work? Ride your bicycle? How about parking your car a half mile from work—or getting off at a bus or subway stop farther away and walking the rest of the way? How about taking the stairs or walking instead of driving to lunch? Better yet, go for a walk at lunchtime and brown-bag a Paleo lunch afterward. You can even keep a portable stair-stepping device and a few small dumbbells in your office. Maybe you have access to a health club or a gym near work where you can take a quick swim, do some weight lifting, or get in a game of racquetball during your lunch hour. When you go to the restroom, take a roundabout route up and down a couple of flights of stairs. Because almost everybody notices an increase in daily energy levels (there is no mid-afternoon slump) within days of starting the Paleo Diet, you will have the energy and spirit for these extra activities. Look for physical activity—lifting, walking, climbing stairs, digging in the garden—wherever you can. Anything extra you can do is better than doing nothing, and all of these little increments add up.

At home, try not to use some of your laborsaving devices. For example, a snowblower gets the job done faster, but unless you're going to use the time saved for exercise later in the day, shoveling the snow would be much better for you. Important note: Beware the "weekend warrior" syndrome. If you have been sedentary, don't charge in with major aerobic exercise all at once. Talk to your doctor and figure out the safest, best way for you to get back in shape.

Increasing Your Activity Level during Leisure Time

During your leisure time, instead of watching a fishing show on TV, go fishing. Instead of watching a football game on TV, go out and throw the football around with your children. Instead of playing games on the computer, go for a walk or a hike or do some gardening. When you go to the beach, don't just sit there; try a bit of swimming, a walk, or maybe even jog in the sand. Leisure-time activities can be enjoyable and still involve exertion. When you go shopping, make sure you do as much walking as possible. Camping trips don't necessarily have to be junk-food feasts involving little or no physical activity. You can enjoy the great outdoors by doing something in it, such as hiking, chopping wood, or swimming. Be creative. Developing a more active life at home and at work will give you a great start in emulating the exercise patterns of our Paleolithic ancestors and will go a long way toward improving your health. Unless you do very strenuous work on the job or at home, however, you will probably need to complement your daily work and leisure activities with a structured exercise program as well.

Structured Exercise Programs

The physical activities of hunter-gatherers most closely resembled those of modern cross-training athletes, in that they were required to do both aerobic and strength activities periodically. Men commonly hunted from one to four days a week, with intervening days of rest. Hunting involved long walks and jogging (up to 10 to 15 miles) to find herd animals; dramatic sprints, jumps, and turns; occasionally violent struggles; and lengthy hikes home carrying the kill. Every two or three days, women routinely gathered; they spent many hours walking to sources of food, water, and wood. Foraging often involved strenuous digging, climbing, and then carrying heavy loads back to camp—usually with an infant or a young child on the woman's hip or back. Other common activities, some physically taxing, included taking care of children, making tools, building shelters, butchering animals, preparing food, and visiting. Dances were a major pastime and could take place several nights a week— often lasting for hours. The overall activity pattern of these people was cyclic: days of intense physical exertion (both aerobic and resistive) alternated with days of rest and light activity.

These activity patterns suggest that most of us are best adapted to exercise programs that alternate strength and aerobic activities, accompanied by intervening days of rest or low-level activities. As you develop an exercise program, you should keep these concepts in mind. Hard days should be followed by one or more easy days, and strength training (weight lifting) should accompany aerobic training. Although the bottom line is that any exercise is better than no exercise, you will be less susceptible to injury and will obtain superior overall fitness if you can follow these fundamental principles.

Aerobic Training Programs

You may already be fit and exercising regularly. Or you may do sporadic exercise. Or maybe you are overweight, and you hardly ever exercise. What you begin to do now—the amount and intensity of your exercise program—will necessarily depend on your starting point.

In order to gain the minimal health effects of exercise, you will need to accumulate at least *thirty minutes of aerobic activity* (walking, jogging, swimming, cycling, aerobic dance, stair climbing, racquetball, basketball, etc.) of *moderate intensity* on most, and *preferably all, days of the week*. Additional health and functional benefits of physical activity can be achieved by devoting more time to the activity, by increasing the vigor of the activity, or by increasing the number of times per week you exercise.

If you're a beginner, you may not be able to walk for thirty minutes a day, every day, right away. Always listen to your body and increase or decrease your exercise accordingly. If you have a family history of heart disease, are very obese, or have other health problems, you should talk to your doctor or even have a checkup before you begin your exercise program. However, don't use this as an excuse to avoid exercising. *Not* exercising is more hazardous to your health than exercising is. If you feel sore or tired from a day's exercise, take the next day off, just as our hunter-gatherer ancestors would have done. Gradually, as you become more and more fit, you will be able to increase the frequency, intensity, and duration of your exercise program. Your fitness level will generally change more rapidly if you heighten the intensity of exercise, rather than increase the frequency or duration.

The key to any successful aerobic training program is to stick with it. You need to keep it interesting and stimulating. The best way to sabotage an aerobic training program is to walk in boring circles around a track or ride a stationary bicycle in your closet. Personally, I find jogging or walking on hiking trails or little-used dirt roads on the edge of town to be much more stimulating and peaceful than jogging on city streets. I can see birds and wildlife. The terrain and the view are constantly changing, and I don't have to fight traffic. It may take you a little longer to drive to a trailhead or a walking path, but you may find that it's worth it. If you live in a metropolitan area, a large city park may be ideal for walks and jogs. You may prefer swimming or bicycling, or you may be more sociable and prefer the company of others while doing aerobic dance, stair climbing, or stationary bicycling in a health club or a gymnasium. Vary your aerobic activities; take your dog with you; bring a pair of binoculars and look for birds; travel to the park or hiking trails; swim at the ocean or the lake. Don't look at exercise as a form of penance. Make it fun, and make it stimulating.

Strength Training Programs

Strength training should be performed at least twice a week, incorporating a minimum of eight to ten specific exercises that use the major muscle groups of the legs, the trunk, the arms, and the shoulders. You should perform at least one or two sets of eight to twelve repetitions in each set. To minimize the risk of muscle injury, it's a good idea to do plenty of stretching and light calisthenics as a warm-up—the same for aerobic exercise. If you do not have a weight machine or a set of free weights at home, visit your local health club or fitness center to get started. Most health clubs and fitness centers employ knowledgeable personnel who can help you get started and can show you how to lift properly and use the weight machines. Once you figure out the basics, you may want to purchase equipment for your home.

Cross-Train—Just Like Your Paleolithic Ancestors

I encourage you not just to walk or swim or lift weights. Try to incorporate both strength and aerobic activities in your fitness program. This is the way our Paleolithic ancestors did it, and this is the method that will increase your fitness levels most rapidly, while simultaneously preventing injuries. If your legs are sore or tired from walking, then take the next day off or do some weight lifting that emphasizes the muscles of your upper body. Swimming is a wonderful exercise that temporarily neutralizes the force of gravity and allows free movement of the joints and the muscles. Even if walking or jogging is your main aerobic activity, try to swim a few times a month. It will give your body a needed break from jogging's incessant pounding and will allow you to stretch your muscles and joints fully. Using a cross-training machine, bicycling and stationary bicycling, like swimming, can also work wonders in relieving the stress from too much walking or jogging. When you alternate strength activities with various aerobic activities, you will not only speed up the development of fitness, but you will lessen your chances of injury.

. . .

Think of exercise as a luxury, a wonderful, opulent pursuit that is not available to all. It is a miraculous elixir that will brighten your spirits, improve your well-being, and make you feel so much better! Exercise will help you complete and maintain your wonderful new Paleo way of life.

12

Living the Paleo Diet

I have given you the key to the door, but I cannot open it for you. For the first time in your life, you should realize that by eating the diet nature devised for us, you can achieve permanent weight loss and significantly improve your health. All of this can occur without your experiencing continual feelings of hunger.

Humanity's original diet is not prescribed to you by a diet doctor or by governmental recommendations, but rather by more than 2 million years of evolutionary wisdom. This is the diet that every single person on the planet ate a mere 333 generations ago. Paleolithic people had no choice but to follow the Paleo Diet. Refined grains, sugars, salt, dairy products, fatty meats, and processed food simply didn't exist. Unfortunately, from a health and weight perspective, you have a choice. Burgers, fries, and a Coke are just down the block—but so are healthful fruits, vegetables, and lean meats. The choice is yours.

How can you empower yourself? How can you make the correct choice happen every time? Here are a few simple guidelines that will help.

The Right Reasons to Eat

Let's once more follow the course given to us by our hunter-gatherer ancestors. Eat when you are hungry, and stop eating when you are full. Many of us eat for all the wrong reasons.

Food is love. Remember that birthday cake you ate on your special day as a child? It brought you warmth and security—it may

209

have represented your parents' love. Many of us still associate sugary, rich desserts with love and fond childhood memories. That's okay; in fact, food should still be associated with love. But why not try to love yourself, your family, or your friends with some of nature's original loving food, so that by eating, you are also loving your body and making yourself healthy? How about a few rich lobster tails or fresh crab legs, some creamy avocado slices, or a bowl of fresh blackberries topped with almond slices? These foods taste great and make you feel great. Those childhood love foods (cookies, cakes, candy, ice cream, chocolates—you know the rest) are a temporary fix that all too soon will make you feel tired, drowsy, and bloated. How many times do you need to "love yourself" with these foods to know that they always let you down in the long run?

Food is a reward. Remember going out to dinner after high school graduation, your wedding, or getting that new job? You rewarded yourself by eating a great meal—and rightly so. You deserved it, and you still do. However, many of us seek that reward or gratification from our food almost daily. Reward yourself with food, and do it daily, but do it with the delicious bounty of real foods: fruits, vegetables, and lean meats. You will be rewarding not only your psyche but your body as well.

Food relieves boredom. Have you ever sat around on a Friday evening with nothing to do, knowing there is a half gallon of ice cream in the refrigerator? How about an afternoon home alone with some chocolate chip cookies fresh out of the oven? When you adopt the Paleo Diet, these situations will no longer be a problem. You will have a ton of food at home, but it will be fruits, veggies, lean meats, and seafood. Go ahead—get bored all you want, and please eat all you want, because your appetite will tell you when to stop. You could probably eat the entire half gallon of ice cream and the whole plate of cookies, but you will always stop eating when you've had your fill of lean chicken breasts, succulent tiger shrimp, or fresh tangerines. Use these foods to relieve your boredom, and you will find yourself losing weight and taking a new path toward terrific health.

One Day at a Time

If you are like almost everyone on this planet, you probably have never made it through a single day of your life without eating grains, dairy products, legumes, salt, refined sugars, fatty meats, or processed foods and drinks.

Go ahead, try it—just once!

I challenge you to eat nothing but fresh fruits, veggies, and lean meats for a single day. You will not be hungry. Eat as much and as many of these foods as you want—eat until you are full. I can assure you that you will not develop vitamin or mineral deficiencies; on the contrary, you will be luxuriously nourished.

See for yourself—see how you feel when you wake up the next morning.

Follow the Paleo Diet principles all day long for a second day. You can do it. If you get hungry or are tempted, treat yourself to a big bowl of fruit or some cold chicken breasts or any of the wonderful Paleo snacks listed in chapter 9. Monitor your energy level. Do you like waking up feeling positive and energized, looking forward to a bright new day? Do you like the way it feels *not* to have that midmorning or midafternoon slump? Well, this is just the beginning. Most people report these healthful benefits within days of adopting the Paleo Diet.

But the best is yet to come. Your weight will drop rapidly within the first few days, and then you will continue to lose weight until you reach your optimal weight. For some people, this may take a month or two; for those with severe weight problems, six months or more. But the bottom line is that you will continue to lose weight as long as you follow the Paleo Diet principles. If weight loss is your primary goal, then focus on how you would like to look in a month or two. Your confidence will soar as you begin to shed the pounds. Your clothes will begin to fit a bit looser. Good—you are well on your way! People will notice your new svelteness. Use these markers as your personal triumphs. Know that these little victories may take weeks or months but that the battle is won on a daily basis. Try to remember how good each morning feels when you stick with the diet. This is where it counts—day to day. The days become weeks, and the weeks become months, and you will eventually break through and reach your weight-loss goal—whatever it may be.

You may also notice that many health problems you had lived with or ignored for years begin to improve. Your joints are no longer as stiff in the morning, and your sinuses are now beginning to clear. Your skin and hair are becoming softer and less dry. Your heartburn and indigestion have become a thing of the past. And for the first time in years, your constipation or irritable bowel syndrome is gone.

For those with more serious health problems, such as high blood pressure and elevated cholesterol or type 2 diabetes, symptoms may begin to improve within weeks of adopting the Paleo Diet.

You have the key to unlock the door of good health with humanity's original diet. What better reason to permanently adopt the Paleo Diet than to prevent heart disease, type 2 diabetes, hypertension, or other symptoms of metabolic syndrome. Play it smart. Remove the known or suspected causes of metabolic syndrome from your diet. When you do, you will also lower your risk of developing many types of cancer as well.

The choice is yours. The risks are nil, the benefits are many. Eat your fill to health and the right weight. And don't forget to enjoy!

APPENDIX A

Acid-Base Values of Common Foods
(100-gram portions)

Acid Foods (1 Values)		Alkaline Foods (2 Values)	
Grains		*Fruits*	
Brown rice	+12.5	Raisins	−21.0
Rolled oats	+10.7	Black currants	−6.5
Spaghetti	+6.5	Bananas	−5.5
Egg noodles	+6.4	Apricots	−4.8
Cornflakes	+6.0	Kiwi fruit	−4.1
White rice	+4.6	Cherries	−3.6
Rye bread	+4.1	Pears	−2.9
Mixed wheat bread	+3.8	Pineapple	−2.7
White bread	+3.7	Peaches	−2.4
		Apples	−2.2
Dairy Foods		Watermelon	−1.9
Parmesan cheese	+34.2	*Vegetables*	
Processed cheese	+28.7	Spinach	−14.0
Hard cheeses	+19.2	Celery	−5.2
Gouda cheese	+18.6	Carrots	−4.9
Camembert cheese	+14.6	Zucchini	−4.6
Cottage cheese	+8.7	Cauliflower	−4.0
Whole milk	+0.7	Potatoes	−4.0
Legumes		Radish	−3.7
Peanuts	+8.3	Eggplant	−3.4
Lentils	+3.5	Tomatoes	−3.1
Peas	+1.2	Lettuce	−2.5
Meat, Fish, Eggs		Chicory	−2.0
Trout	+10.8	Leeks	−1.8
Turkey	+9.9	Onions	−1.5
Chicken	+8.7	Mushrooms	−1.4
Eggs	+8.1	Green peppers	−1.4
Pork	+7.9	Broccoli	−1.2
Beef	+7.8	Cucumber	−0.8
Cod	+7.1		
Herring	+7.0		

APPENDIX B

Comparison of the Total Fat in Domestic and Wild Meats

Fatty Domestic Meat	% Fat	Grams of Saturated Fat
Pork chop	51	4.80
T-bone beefsteak	66	9.08
Lamb chop	75	9.95
Chicken thigh	58	4.33
average = 62.5		7.04

Wild meat	% Fat	Grams of Saturated Fat
Bison roast	16	0.91
Antelope roast	17	0.97
Moose roast	7	0.29
Deer roast	19	1.25
average = 14.8		0.86

APPENDIX C

Practical Implementation of Parts of the Paleo Diet on a Global Scale

In this book, I've traced agricultural "progress," and we've seen that the key to restoring our health and losing weight is to replace our modern processed foods with fresh fruits, vegetables, lean meats, and seafood. In the United States and other Western countries, this is very easy to do. We can grow our own vegetables and fruits or buy them year round at the supermarket. Thanks to global air transportation and greenhouses, we can get fresh peaches in February and strawberries in December. We can get shrimp from Tahiti in Minnesota, buy Colorado-raised buffalo meat in Hawaii, and find Alaskan salmon in Nebraska.

The only limiting factor is cost. Fresh fruits and vegetables cost more than beans and white rice. Lean pork tenderloin and turkey breasts are more expensive than potatoes and bread. The starchy foods of the Agricultural Revolution are the world's cheap foods. Grains, legumes, and tubers are the starchy foods that have let our planet's population balloon to more than 6 billion. They're also the foods that have enabled us to grotesquely fatten our livestock in feedlots to satisfy our craving for fatty meats. They've allowed us to pollute our food supply with billions of tons of sugar and high-fructose corn syrup. They're also the foods responsible for destroying the balance of omega 6 and omega 3 fats in our diet. Without them, the world could probably support one-tenth or less of our present population; without agriculture's cheap starchy staples, it is no exaggeration to say that billions of people worldwide would starve.

It is unfortunate that for most of the world's people the diet to which they are genetically adapted now lies beyond their financial

reach. The foods decreed by our genetic heritage and the foods
we all ate before the Agricultural Revolution have now become the
elite foods of wealthy, privileged countries.

However, there are many immediate practical steps that could
be taken to improve the nutritional quality of the world's food supply and make everyday diets more like those of our Paleolithic
ancestors.

Healthier Livestock

Cereal grains are an inferior food for livestock as well as for humans.
Many of our health problems related to overconsumption of saturated fats and omega 6 fats are directly attributable to the practice
of feeding grain to livestock. Today, 70 percent of the U.S. grain
harvest is fed to cattle, but there is no pressing need to do this. In
modern beef production, cattle generally spend the first half of
their lives grazing on pastureland or rangeland. They typically receive commercial cereal feeds during the second half of their lives.
If we didn't confine cattle to feedlots and essentially force-feed
them cereal grains, we could produce a healthier meat product by
simply allowing these animals the freedom to graze outdoors all
their lives.

Feeding grain to cattle dilutes the healthful omega 3 fats and
increases the omega 6 fats. It also produces an obese animal that
may have as much as 25 to 30 percent of its body weight as fat.
Three- to 4-inch layers of pure fat lie just below the skin. Fat dominates the abdominal cavity and even infiltrates the muscle tissue.
This infiltration of fat between the muscles, called "marbling," is
one of the major reasons why grain is fed to cattle: cattle producers believe the consumer likes a nicely marbled steak. But a nicely
marbled T-bone steak may contain more than 60 percent of its total
calories as fat. Even lean, grain-fed beef, trimmed of all of its fat,
contains more than twice the fat that is found in pasture-fed cattle
or wild game meat. The predominant type of fat in grain-fattened
cows is saturated fat. A 100-gram serving of a fatty T-bone steak
gives you 9 grams of saturated fat. The same serving of a lean steak
from a pasture-fed cow gives you only 1.3 grams of saturated fat.

Feeding grain to cattle has a harmful effect on nutrients as
well: cattle fed on pasture alone produce meat that contains five
times more conjugated linoleic acid (CLA) than grain-fed cattle

do. Conjugated linoleic acid is a good type of fat that may be one of our most powerful allies in the war against cancer; in studies of laboratory animals, tiny amounts of CLA have effectively reduced tumor growth. Grass-fed livestock also produce meat that contains four times more vitamin E and selenium than grain-fed animals have. Both vitamin E and selenium are powerful antioxidants that protect us from cancer and heart disease.

Basically, feeding grain to cattle takes a good, healthful food—lean meat—and turns it into a less nutritious, fatty food that has a high potential for impairing our health. It's also very wasteful. Most of the excess fat from cows that produce marbled meat is ultimately trimmed away and discarded during the butchering process. Why are we feeding grain to our livestock to make them fat and then throwing away much of the fat just to get an end product—fatty meat—that is less healthful than the original lean meat we started with? It makes little sense. A better approach to raising our cattle, from both health and ecological viewpoints, would be simply to eliminate grain feeding altogether. Many of the beef producers in Australia and Argentina have taken this approach, with a resounding note of approval from the consumer.

Resources

Recommended Web Sites

Loren Cordain's Paleo Diet Web site
www.thepaleodiet.com

Loren Cordain's Dietary Cure for Acne Web site
http://www.dietaryacnecure.com/

Robb Wolf's Web site
http://robbwolf.com/

Don Wiss's comprehensive Paleo Web site
http://paleodiet.com/

Recommended Books

Cordain, Loren. *The Dietary Cure for Acne.* Fort Collins, CO: Paleo Diet Enterprises LLC, 2006.

Cordain, Loren, and Joe Friel. *The Paleo Diet for Athletes: A Nutritional Formula for Peak Athletic Performance.* Emmaus, PA: Rodale Press, 2005.

Cordain, Loren, Nell Stephenson, and Lorrie Cordain. *The Paleo Diet Cookbook: More Than 150 Recipes for Paleo Breakfasts, Lunches, Dinners, Snacks, and Beverages.* Hoboken, NJ: John Wiley & Sons, 2011.

Suppliers of Paleo-Related Foods

Paleo Brands
http://www.paleobrands.com/

Suppliers of Game Meats

Broken Arrow Ranch
3296 Junction Highway
Ingram, TX 78025
(800) 962-4263
www.brokenarrowranch.com

Exotic Meat Market
130 Walnut Avenue, Unit A-18
Perris, CA 92571
951-345-4623
http://exoticmeatmarket.com/

Exotic Meats USA
1330 Capita Blvd.
Reno, NV 89502
(800) 444-5687
http://www.exoticmeatsandmore.com/

Game Sales International
P.O. Box 7719
Loveland, CO 80537
(800) 729-2090
www.gamesalesintl.com

Grande Natural Meat
P.O. Box 10
Del Norte, Colorado 81132
(888) 338-4581
www.elkusa.com

Hills Foods Ltd.
Unit 130 Glacier Street
Coquitlam, British Columbia
Canada V3K 5Z6
(604) 472-1500
www.hillsfoods.com

Mount Royal Game Meat
3902 N. Main
Houston, TX 77009
(800) 730-3337
www.mountroyal.com

Polarica
105 Quint Street
San Francisco, CA 94124
(800) 426-3872
www.polarica.com

Suppliers of Pasture- and Grass-Produced Meats, Eggs and Dairy

Jo Robinson's comprehensive listing of pasture and grass-fed meats,
   eggs, and dairy in the U.S. and Canada
http://www.eatwild.com/

George Bass's free-range eggs:
The Country Hen
P.O. Box 333
Hubbardston, MA 01452
Phone: (978) 928-5333
countryhen.com

Bibliography

Adachi J, Hasegawa M. Improved dating of the human/chimpanzee separation in the mitochondrial DNA tree: heterogeneity among amino acid sites. *J Mol Evol* 1995;40:622–628.

Adams PB, Lawson S, Sanigorski A, Sinclair AJ. Arachidonic acid to eicosapentaenoic acid ratio in blood correlates positively with clinical symptoms of depression. *Lipids* 1996;31:S157–S161.

Adebamowo CA, Spiegelman D, Berkey CS, Danby FW, Rockett HH, Colditz GA, Willett WC, Holmes MD. Milk consumption and acne in teenaged boys. *J Am Acad Dermatol* 2008;58(5):787–793.

Adebamowo CA, Spiegelman D, Berkey CS, Danby FW, Rockett HH, Colditz GA, Willett WC, Holmes MD. Milk consumption and acne in adolescent girls. *Dermatol Online J* 2006;12(4):1.

Adebamowo CA, Spiegelman D, Danby FW, Frazier AL, Willett WC, Holmes MD. High school dietary dairy intake and teenage acne. *J Am Acad Dermatol* 2005;52(2):207–214.

Aiello LC, Wheeler P. The expensive tissue hypothesis. *Curr Anthropol* 1995;36: 199–222.

Ainsleigh HG. Beneficial effects of sun exposure on cancer mortality. *Prev Med* 1993;22:132–140.

Aizawa H, Niimura M. Elevated serum insulin-like growth factor-1 (IGF-1) levels in women with postadolescent acne. *J Dermatol* 1995;22:249–252.

——— . Mild insulin resistance during oral glucose tolerance test (OGTT) in women with acne. *J Dermatol* 1996;23:526–529.

Albanes D, Jones DV, Schatzkin A, Micozzi MS, Taylor PR. Adult stature and risk of cancer. *Can Res* 1988;48:1658–1662.

Albert CM, Hennekens CH, O'Donnell CJ, Ajani UA, Carey VJ, Willett WC, Ruskin JN, Manson JE. Fish consumption and risk of sudden cardiac death. *JAMA* 1998;279:23–28.

American Heart Association. *2000 Heart and Stroke Statistical Update.* Dallas, TX: American Heart Association, 1999.

Anderson GH. Dietary patterns vs. dietary recommendations: identifying the gaps for complex carbohydrate. *Crit Rev Food Sci Nutr* 1994;5&6:435–440.

Antonios TT, MacGregor GA. Deleterious effects of salt intake other than effects on blood pressure. *Clin Exp Pharmacol Physiol* 1995;22:180–184.

Appel LJ, Moore TJ, Obarzanek E, Vollmer WM, Svetkey LP, Sacks FM, Bray GA, Vogt TM, Cutler JA, Windhauser MM, Lin PH, Karanja N. A clinical trial of the effects of dietary patterns on blood pressure. *N Engl J Med* 1997;336: 1117–1124.

Armelagos GJ. Human evolution and the evolution of disease. *Ethn Dis* 1991;1: 21–25.

Attia N, Tamborlane WV, Heptulla R, Maggs D, Grozman A, Sherwin RS, Caprio S. The metabolic syndrome and insulin-like growth factor I regulation in adolescent obesity. *J Clin Endocrinol Metab* 1998;83:1467–1471.

Baaregaard A. Dental conditions and nutrition among natives in Greenland. *Oral Surg, Oral Med, Oral Pathol* 1949;2:995–1007.

Baba NH, Sawaya S, Torbay N, Habbal Z, Azar S, Hashim SA. High protein vs. high carbohydrate hypoenergetic diet for the treatment of obese hyperinsulinemic subjects. *Int J Obes Relat Metab Disord* 1999;23:1202–1206.

Balam G, Gurri F. A physiological adaptation to undernutrition. *Ann Hum Biol* 1994;21:483–489.

Bang O, Dyerberg J. Lipid metabolism and ischemic heart disease in Greenland Eskimos. *Adv Nutr Res* 1980;3:1–22.

Barkeling B, Rossner S, Bjorvell H. Effects of a high-protein meal (meat) and a high-carbohydrate meal (vegetarian) on satiety measured by automated computerized monitoring of subsequent food intake, motivation to eat and food preferences. *Int J Obes* 1990;14:743–751.

Barzel US. The skeleton as an ion exchange system: implications for the role of acid-base imbalance in the genesis of osteoporosis. *J Bone Min Res* 1995;10: 1431–1436.

Bershad S, Poulin YP, Berson DS, Sabean J, Brodell RT, Shalita AR, Kakita L, Tanghetti E, Leyden J, Webster GF, Miller BH. Topical retinoids in the treatment of acne vulgaris. *Cutis* 1999;64(suppl 2):8–20.

Bicchieri MG (ed.). *Hunters and Gatherers Today.* New York: Holt, Rinehart and Winston, 1972.

Binoux M, Gourmelen M. Statural development parallels IGF I levels in subjects of constitutionally variant stature. *Acta Endocrinol* 1987;114: 524–530.

Bitzer M, Feldkaemper M, Schaeffel F. Visually induced changes in components of the retinoic acid system in fundal layers of the chick. *Exp Eye Res* 2000;70: 97–106.

Black HS, Thornby JI, Gerguis J, Lenger W. Influence of dietary omega-6, -3 fatty acid sources on the initiation and promotion stages of photocarcinogenesis. *Photochem Photobiol* 1992;56:195–199.

Blair R, Misir R. Biotin bioavailability from protein supplements and cereal grains for growing broiler chickens. *Int J Vit Nutr Res* 1989;59:55–58.

Block G, Patterson B, Subar A. Fruit, vegetables, and cancer prevention: a review of the epidemiological evidence. *Nutr Cancer* 1992;18:1–29.

Blum WF, Albertsson-Wikland K, Rosberg S, Ranke MB. Serum levels of insulin-like growth factor I (IGF-I) and IGF binding protein 3 reflect spontaneous growth hormone secretion. *J Clin Endocrinol Metab* 1993;76:1610–1616.

Blumenschine RJ. Carcass consumption sequences and the archaeological distinction of scavenging and hunting. *J Hum Evol* 1986;15:639–659.

Blumenschine RJ, Cavallo JA. Scavenging and human evolution. *Sci Am* 1992;267: 90–96.

Blumenschine RJ, Madrigal TC. Variability in long bone marrow yields of East African ungulates and its zooarchaeological implications. *J Archaeo Sci* 1993;20:555–587.

Boeda E, Geneste JM, Griggo C, Mercier N, Muhesen S, Reyss JL, Taha A, Valladas H. A Levallois point embedded in the vertebra of a wild ass (*Equus africanus*): hafting, projectiles and Mousterian hunting weapons. *Antiquity* 1999;73:394–402.

Boutton TW, Lynott MJ, Bumsted MP. Stable carbon isotopes and the study of prehistoric diet. *Crit Rev Food Sci Nutr* 1991;30:373–385.

Brand-Miller JC, Holt SHA. Australian aboriginal plant foods: a consideration of their nutritional composition and health implications. *Nut Res Rev* 1998;11: 5–23.

Breslow RA, Hallfrisch J, Guy DG, Crawley B, Goldberg AP. The importance of dietary protein in healing pressure ulcers. *J Am Geriatr Soc* 1993;41: 357–362.

Brismar K, Fernqvist-Forbes E, Wahren J, Hall K. Effect of insulin on the hepatic production of insulin-like growth factor-binding protein-1 (IGFBP-1), IGFBP-3, and IGF-1 in insulin dependent diabetes. *J Clin Endocrinol Metab* 1994;79:872–878.

Brouwer IA, Katan MB, Zock PL. Dietary alpha-linolenic acid is associated with reduced risk of fatal coronary heart disease, but increased prostate cancer risk: a meta-analysis. *J Nutr* 2004;134(4):919–922.

Bruning PF, Bonfrer JM, van Noord PA, Hart AA, de Jong-Bakker M, Nooijen WJ. Insulin resistance and breast cancer risk. *Int J Cancer* 1992;52: 511–516.

Bunn HT, Kroll EM. Systematic butchery by Plio/Pleistocene hominids at Olduvai Gorge, Tanzania. *Curr Anthropol* 1986;27:431–452.

Burch ES, Ellanna LJ (eds.). *Key Issues in Hunter-Gatherer Research*. Oxford, UK: Berg Publishers, 1994.

Camacho-Hubner C, Woods KA, Miraki-Moud F, Hindmarsh PC, Clark AJ, Hansson Y, Johnston A, Baxter RC, Savage MO. Effects of recombinant human insulin-like growth factor I (IGF-I) therapy on the growth hormone-IGF system of a patient with a partial IGF-I gene deletion. *J Clin Endocrinol Metab* 1999;84:1611–1616.

Cameron A, Jones J, Elliott B, Gorman L. *The L.L. Bean Game and Fish Cookbook*. New York: Random House, 1983.

Canned tuna. *Consumer Reports* 1992(February);103–114.

Caprio S. Differences between African American and white girls in the insulin-like growth factor-I and the binding proteins: importance of insulin resistance and hyperinsulinemia. *J Pediatr* 1999;135:270–271.

Carayol M, Grosclaude P, Delpierre C. Prospective studies of dietary alpha-linolenic acid intake and prostate cancer risk: a meta-analysis. *Cancer Causes Control* 2010;21(3):347–355.

Cary OJ, Locke C, Cookson JB. Effect of alterations of dietary sodium on the severity of asthma in men. *Thorax* 1993;48:714–718.

Catlin, G. *Letters and Notes on the Manners, Customs, and Conditions of North American Indians*. New York: Dover Publications, 1973.

Chambers JC, Obeid OA, Refsum H, Ueland P, Hackett D, Hooper J, Turner RM, Thompson SG, Kooner JS. Plasma homocysteine concentrations and risk of coronary heart disease in UK Indian Asian and European men. *Lancet* 2000;355:523–527.

Chan JM. Nutrition and acid-base metabolism. *Fed Proc* 1981;40:2423–2428.

Chanmugam P, Boudreau M, Hwang DH. Differences in the omega 3 fatty acid contents in pond-reared and wild fish and shellfish. *J Food Sci* 1986;51: 1556–1557.

Chew SJ, Balakrishnan V. Myopia produced in young chicks by intermittent minimal form visual deprivation—can spectacles cause myopia? *Singapore Med J* 1992;33:489–492.

Clark LC, Combs GF Jr, Turnbull BW, Slate EH, Chalker DK, Chow J, Davis LS, Glover RA, Graham GF, Gross EG, Krongrad A, Lesher JL Jr, Park HK, Sanders BB Jr, Smith CL, Taylor JR. Effects of selenium supplementation for cancer prevention in patients with carcinoma of the skin. A randomized controlled trial. Nutritional Prevention of Cancer Study Group. *JAMA* 1996;276:1957–1963.

Cleave TL. *The Saccharine Disease*. Bristol: John Wright & Sons, 1974.

Cockburn A. Where did our infectious diseases come from? The evolution of infectious disease. *Ciba Found Symp* 1977;49:103–112.

Cohen MN. The significance of long-term changes in human diet and food economy. In Harris M, Ross EB (eds.), *Food and Evolution. Toward a*

Theory of Human Food Habits, Philadelphia: Temple University Press, 1987, pp. 261–283.

Cohen MN, Armelagos GJ. *Paleopathology at the Origins of Agriculture.* New York: Academic Press, 1984.

Cordain L. Dietary implications for the development of acne: a shifting paradigm. In Bedlow J (ed.), *U.S. Dermatology Review II.* London: Touch Briefings Publications, 2006.

Cordain L. Implications for the role of diet in acne. *Semin Cutan Med Surg* 2005;24(2):84–91.

Cordain L. Paleodiet and Paleolithic Nutrition: The Cordain Files. www .beyondveg.com/cat/paleodiet/index.shtml.

————. Atherogenic potential of peanut oil–based monounsaturated fatty acids diets. *Lipids* 1998;33:229–230.

————. Cereal grains: humanity's double-edged sword. *World Rev Nutr Diet* 1999;84:19–73.

Cordain L, Brand-Miller J, Eaton SB, Mann N. Reply to SC Cunnane. *Am J Clin Nutr* 2000;72:1585–1586.

————. Macronutrient estimations in hunter-gatherer diets. *Am J Clin Nutr* 2000;72:1589–1590.

Cordain L, Brand-Miller J, Eaton SB, Mann N, Holt SH, Speth JD. Plant-animal subsistence ratios and macronutrient energy estimations in worldwide hunter-gatherer diets. *Am J Clin Nutr* 2000;71:682–692.

Cordain L, Bryan ED, Melby CL, Smith MJ. Influence of moderate daily wine consumption upon body weight regulation and metabolism in healthy, free living males. *J Am Coll Nutr* 1997;16:134–139.

Cordain L, Eades MR, Eades MD. Hyperinsulinemic diseases of civilization: more than just Syndrome X. *Comp Biochem Physiol A Mol Integr Physiol* 2003;136(1):95–112

Cordain L, Eaton SB, Brand-Miller J, Lindeberg S, Jensen C. An evolutionary analysis of the aetiology and pathogenesis of juvenile-onset myopia. *Acta Ophthalmol Scand* 2002;80(2):125–135.

Cordain L, Eaton SB, Brand-Miller J, Mann N, Hill K. The paradoxical nature of hunter-gatherer diets: Meat based, yet non-atherogenic. *Eur J Clin Nutr* in press.

Cordain L, Eaton SB, Sebastian A, Mann N, Lindeberg S, Watkins BA, O'Keefe JH, Brand-Miller J. Origins and evolution of the Western diet: health implications for the 21st century. *Am J Clin Nutr* 2005;81(2): 341–354.

Cordain L, Gotshall RW. Compiled ethnographic observations of the aerobic fitness, strength and body composition of unacculturated humans. *Med Sci Sports Exerc* 1999;31:S213.

Cordain L, Gotshall RW, Eaton SB. Evolutionary aspects of exercise. *World Rev Nutr Diet* 1997;81:49–60.

Cordain L, Gotshall RW, Eaton SB, Eaton SB III. Physical activity, energy expenditure and fitness: an evolutionary perspective. *Int J Sport Med* 1998;19: 328–335.

Cordain L, Lindeberg S, Hurtado M, Hill K, Eaton SB, Brand-Miller J. Acne vulgaris: a disease of Western civilization. *Arch Dermatol* 2002;138(12): 1584–1590.

Cordain L, Martin C, Florant G, Watkins BA. The fatty acid composition of muscle, brain, marrow and adipose tissue in elk: evolutionary implications for human dietary lipid requirements. *World Rev Nutr Diet* 1998;83:225.

Cordain L, Melby CL, Hamamoto AE, O'Neill S, Cornier MA, Barakat HA, Israel RG, Hill JO. Influence of moderate chronic wine consumption on insulin sensitivity and other correlates of syndrome X in moderately obese women. *Metabolism* 2000;49:1473–1478.

Cordain L, Miller J, Mann N. Scant evidence of periodic starvation among hunter-gatherers. *Diabetologia* 1999;42:383–384.

Cordain L, Toohey L, Smith MJ, Hickey MS. Modulation of immune function by dietary lectins in rheumatoid arthritis. *Br J Nutr* 2000;83:207–217.

Cordain L, Watkins BA, Florant G, Kehler M, Rogers L. A detailed fatty acid analysis of selected tissues in elk, mule deer, and antelope. *FASEB J* 1999:13: A887.

Cordain L, Watkins BA, Florant GL, Kehler M, Rogers L, Li Y. Fatty acid analysis of wild ruminant tissues: evolutionary implications for reducing diet-related chronic disease. *Eur J Clin Nutr* 2001;56:1–11.

Cordain L, Watkins BA, Mann NJ. Fatty acid composition and energy density of foods available to African hominids: evolutionary implications for human brain development. *World Rev Nutr Diet* 2001;90:144–161.

Crawford MA, Bloom M, Broadhurst CL, Schmidt WF, Cunnane SC, Galli C, Gehbremeskel K, Linseisen F, Lloyd-Smith J, Parkington J. Evidence for the unique function of docosahexaenoic acid during the evolution of the modern hominid brain. *Lipids* 1999;34:s39–s47.

Crawford MA, Gale MM, Woodford MH, Casped NM. Comparative studies on fatty acid composition of wild and domestic meat. *Int J Biochem* 1970;1: 295–305.

Crawford MA, Sinclair AJ. The long chain metabolites of linoleic and linolenic acids in liver and brains of herbivores and carnivores. *Comp Biochem Physiol* 1976;54B:395–401.

Crovetti R, Porrini M, Santangelo A, Testolin G. The influence of thermic effect of food on satiety. *Eur J Clin Nutr* 1998;52:482–488.

Cunliffe WJ, Cotteril JA. The acnes: clinical features, pathogenesis and treatment. In Rook A (ed.), *Major Problems in Dermatology*. Philadelphia: WB Saunders, 1975, vol. 6, pp. 13–14.

Cusin I, Rohner-Jeanrenaud F, Terrettaz J, Jeanrenaud B. Hyperinsulinemia and its impact on obesity and insulin resistance. *Int J Obes Relat Metab Disord* 1992;16(suppl 4):S1–S11.

Dagnelie PC, van Dusseldorp M, van Staveren WA, Hautvast JG. Effects of macrobiotic diets on linear growth in infants and children until 10 years of age. *Eur J Clin Nutr* 1994;48(supp 1):S103–S112.

Dauncey MJ, Bingham SA. Dependence of 24 h energy expenditure in man on the composition of the nutrient intake. *Br J Nutr* 1983;50:1–13.

Davidson PW, Myers GJ, Cox C, Axtell C, Shamlaye C, Sloane-Reeves J, Cernichiari E, Needham L, Choi A, Wang Y, Berlin M, Clarkson TW. Effects of prenatal and postnatal methylmercury exposure from fish consumption on neurodevelopment: outcomes at 66 months of age in the Seychelles Child Development Study. *JAMA* 1998;280:701–707.

Daviglus ML, Stamler J, Orencia AJ, Dyer AR, Liu K, Greenland P, Walsh MK, Morris D, Shekelle RB. Fish consumption and the 30-year risk of fatal myocardial infarction. *N Engl J Med* 1997;336:1046–1053.

de Heinzelin J, Clark JD, White T, Hart W, Renne P, WoldeGabriel G, Beyene Y, Vrba E. Environment and behavior of 2.5-million-year-old Bouri hominids. *Science* 1999;284:625–629.

de Lorgeril M, Salen P, Martin JL, Monjaud I, Delaye J, Mamelle N. Mediterranean diet, traditional risk factors, and the rate of cardiovascular complications after myocardial infarction: final report of the Lyon Diet Heart Study. *Circulation* 1999;99:779–785.

Denton D. *The Hunger for Salt*. New York: Springer-Verlag, 1984.

Deplewski D, Rosenfield RL. Growth hormone and insulin-like growth factors have different effects on sebaceous cell growth and differentiation. *Endocrinology* 1999;140:4089–4094.

Devine A, Criddle RA, Dick IM, Kerr DA, Prince RL. A longitudinal study of the effect of sodium and calcium intakes on regional bone density in postmenopausal women. *Am J Clin Nutr* 1995;62:740–745.

DeVries A. *Primitive Man and His Food*. Chicago: Chandler Book Company, 1952.

Dhiman TR, Anand GR, Satter LD, Pariza MW. Conjugated linoleic acid content of milk from cows fed different diets. *J Dairy Sci* 1999;82:2146–2156.

Diamond J. The worst mistake in the history of the human race. *Discover* 1987(May):64–66.

Dietary supplementation with n-3 polyunsaturated fatty acids and vitamin E after myocardial infarction: results of the GISSI-Prevenzione trial.

Gruppo Italiano per lo Studio della Sopravvivenza nell'Infarto mio-cardico. *Lancet* 1999;354:447–455.

Dirlewanger M, Schneiter P, Jequier E, Tappy L. Effects of fructose on hepatic glucose metabolism in humans. *Am J Physiol Endocrinol Metab* 2000;279: E907–E911.

Dohan FC, Grasberger JC. Relapsed schizophrenics: early discharge from the hospital after cereal-free, milk-free diet. *Am J Psychiatry* 1973;130: 685–688.

Donnelly J, Pronk NP, Jacobsen DJ, Pronk SJ, Jakicic JM. Effects of a very-low-calorie diet and physical-training regimens on body composition and resting metabolic rate in obese females. *Am J Clin Nutr* 1991; 54:56–61.

Douglas JWB, Ross JM, Simpson HR. The ability and attainment of short-sighted pupils. *J R Stat Soc Series A (Gen)* 1967;130:479–504.

Dreon DM, Fernstrom HA, Miller B, Krauss RM. Low-density lipoprotein sub-class patterns and lipoprotein response to a reduced-fat diet in men. *FASEB J* 1994;8:121–126.

Dreon DM, Fernstrom HA, Williams PT, Krauss RM. A very low-fat diet is not associated with improved lipoprotein profiles in men with a predomi-nance of large, low-density lipoproteins. *Am J Clin Nutr* 1999;69: 411–418.

——— . Reduced LDL particle size in children consuming a very-low-fat diet is related to parental LDL-subclass patterns. *Am J Clin Nutr* 2000;71:1611–1616.

Duckett SK, Wagner DG, Yates LD, Dolezal HG, May SG. Effects of time on feed on beef nutrient composition. *J Anim Sci* 1993;71:2079–2088.

Dwyer J, Foulkes E, Evans M, Ausman L. Acid/alkaline ash diets: time for assessment and change. *J Am Diet Assoc* 1985;85:841–845.

Eaton SB, Cordain L, Lindeberg S. Evolutionary health promotion: a consid-eration of common counterarguments. *Prev Med* 2002;34(2):119–123.

Eaton SB, Eaton SB III, Sinclair AJ, Cordain L, Mann NJ. Dietary intake of long-chain polyunsaturated fatty acids during the Paleolithic. *World Rev Nutr Diet* 1998;83:12–23.

Eaton SB, Konner M. Paleolithic nutrition. A consideration of its nature and current implications. *N Engl J Med* 1985;312:283–289.

Eaton SB, Konner M, Shostak M. Stone Agers in the fast lane: chronic degen-erative diseases in evolutionary perspective. *Am J Med* 1988;84:739–749.

Eaton SB, Shostak M, Konner M. The first fitness formula. In *The Paleolithic Prescription*. New York: Harper & Row, pp. 168–199.

Eaton SB, Strassman BI, Nesse RM, Neel JV, Ewald PW, Williams GC, Weder AB, Eaton SB 3rd, Lindeberg S, Konner MJ, Mysterud I, Cordain L. Evo-lutionary health promotion. *Prev Med* 2002;34(2):109–118.

Ercan N, Gannon MC, Nuttall FQ. Effect of added fat on the plasma glucose and insulin response to ingested potato given in various combinations as two meals in normal individuals. *Diabetes Care* 1994;17(12):1453–1459.

Etling K. The wild diet. *Outdoor Life* magazine 1992(August):52–64.

Evans TRJ, Kaye SB. Retinoids: present role and future potential. *Br J Cancer* 1999;80:1–8.

Evershed RP, Payne S, Sherratt AG, Copley MS, Coolidge J, Urem-Kotsu D, et al. Earliest date for milk use in the Near East and southeastern Europe linked to cattle herding. *Nature* 2008;455(7212):528–531.

Ezzo JA, Larsen CS, Burton JH. Elemental signatures of human diets from the Georgia Bight. *Am J Phys Anthropol* 1995;98:471–481.

Falsetti L, Eleftheriou GI. Hyperinsulinemia in the polycystic ovary syndrome: a clinical endocrine and echographic study in 240 patients. *Gynecol Endocrinol* 1996;10:319–326.

Feldkaemper MP, Neacsu I, Schaeffel F. Insulin acts as a powerful stimulator of axial myopia in chicks. *Invest Ophthalmol Vis Sci* 2009;50(1):13–23.

Ferry RJ, Cerri RW, Cohen P. Insulin-like growth factor binding proteins: new proteins, new functions. *Horm Res* 1999;51:53–67.

Feskens EJ, Bowles CH, Kromhout D. Inverse association between fish intake and risk of glucose intolerance in normoglycemic elderly men and women. *Diabetes Care* 1991;14:935–941.

Flegal KM, Carroll MD, Ogden CL, Curtin LR. Prevalence and trends in obesity among US adults, 1999–2008. *JAMA* 2010;303(3):235–241

Foster-Powell K, Brand-Miller J. International tables of glycemic index. *Am J Clin Nutr* 1995;62:871s–893s.

Franceschi S, Favero A. The role of energy and fat in cancers of the breast and colon-rectum in a southern European population. *Ann Oncol* 1999;10(suppl 6):61–63.

Frassetto LA, Morris RC, Sebastian A. Potassium bicarbonate reduces urinary nitrogen excretion in postmenopausal women. *J Clin Endocrinol Metab* 1997; 82:254–259.

Frassetto LA, Todd KM, Morris RC, Sebastian A. Estimation of net endogenous noncarbonic acid production in humans from diet potassium and protein contents. *Am J Clin Nutr* 1998;68:576–583.

Freyre EA, Rebaza RM, Sami DA, Lozada CP. The prevalence of facial acne in Peruvian adolescents and its relation to their ethnicity. *J Adolesc Health* 1998; 22:480–484.

Gabunia L, Vekua A, Lordkipanidze D, Swisher CC III, Ferring R, Justus A, Nioradze M, Tvalchrelidze M, Anton SC, Bosinski G, Joris O, Lumley MA, Majsuradze G, Mouskhelishvili A. Earliest Pleistocene hominid cranial remains from Dmanisi, Republic of Georgia: taxonomy, geological setting, and age. *Science* 2000;288:1019–1025.

Gannon MC, Nuttall FQ, Westphal SA, Fang S, Ercan-Fang N. Acute metabolic response to high-carbohydrate, high-starch meals compared with moderate-carbohydrate, low-starch meals in subjects with type 2 diabetes. *Diabetes Care* 1998;21:1619–1626.

Garcia-Menaya JM, Gonzalo-Garijo MA, Moneo I, Fernandez B, Garcia-Gonzalez F, Moreno F. A 17-kDa allergen detected in pine nuts. *Allergy* 2000;55: 291–293.

Gardiner PA. Dietary treatment of myopia in children. *Lancet* 1958;1:1152–1155.

Gardner CD, Fortmann SP, Krauss RM. Association of small low-density lipoprotein particles with the incidence of coronary artery disease in men and women. *JAMA* 1996;276:875–881.

Gardner CD, Kraemer HC. Monounsaturated versus polyunsaturated dietary fat and serum lipids. A meta-analysis. *Arterioscler Thromb Vasc Biol* 1995;15: 1917–1927.

Garland CF, Garland FC, Gorham ED. Rising trends in melanoma. An hypothesis concerning sunscreen effectiveness. *Ann Epidemiol* 1993;3:103–110.

————— . Calcium and vitamin D. Their potential roles in colon and breast cancer prevention. *Ann NY Acad Sci* 1999;889: 107–119.

Garland FC, Garland CF, Gorham ED, Young JF. Geographic variation in breast cancer mortality in the United States: A hypothesis involving exposure to solar radiation. *Prev Med* 1990;19:614–622.

George R, Bhopal R. Fat composition of free living and farmed sea species: implications for human diet and sea-farming techniques. *Br Food J* 1995;97: 19–22.

Ghafoorunissa. Requirements of dietary fats to meet nutritional needs & prevent the risk of atherosclerosis—an Indian perspective. *Indian J Med Res* 1998;108:191–202.

Gielkens HA, Verkijk M, Lam WF, Lamers CB, Masclee AA. Effects of hyperglycemia and hyperinsulinemia on satiety in humans. *Metabolism* 1998;47: 321–324.

Gill ZP, Perks CM, Newcomb PV, Holly JM. Insulin-like growth factor–binding protein (IGFBP-3) predisposes breast cancer cells to programmed cell death in a non-IGF-dependent manner. *J Biol Chem* 1997;272: 25602–25607.

Giovannucci E. Insulin-like growth factor-I and binding protein-3 and risk of cancer. *Horm Res* 1999;51(suppl S3):34–41.

————— . Tomatoes, tomato-based products, lycopene, and cancer: review of the epidemiologic literature. *J Natl Cancer Inst* 1999;91:317–331.

Giovannucci E, Stampfer MJ, Colditz GA, Rimm EB, Trichopoulos D, Rosner BA, Speizer FE, Willett WC. Folate, methionine, and alcohol intake and risk of colorectal adenoma. *J Natl Cancer Inst* 1993;85:875–883.

Gotshall RW, Mickelborough TD, Cordain L. Dietary salt restriction improves pulmonary function in exercise-induced asthma. *Med Sci Sports Exerc* 2000; 32:1815–1819.

Gourmelen M, Le Bouc Y, Girard F, Binoux M. Serum levels of insulin-like growth factor (IGF) and IGF binding proteins in constitutionally tall children and adolescents. *J Clin Endocrinol Metab* 1984;59:1197–1203.

Gray JP. A corrected ethnographic atlas. *World Cultures J* 1999;10:24–85.

Gray R. *Eat Like a Wild Man: 110 Years of Great Sports Afield Recipes.* Minocqua, WI: Willow Creek Press, 1997.

Greenfield HJ. The origins of milk and wool production in the old world. *Curr Anthropol* 1988;29:573–594.

Griffin BA. Lipoprotein atherogenicity: an overview of current mechanisms. *Proc Nutr Soc* 1999;58:163–169.

Gueux E, Azais-Braesco V, Bussiere L, Grolier P, Mazur A, Rayssiguier Y. Effect of magnesium deficiency on triacylglycerol-rich lipoprotein and tissue susceptibility to peroxidation in relation to vitamin E content. *Br J Nutr* 1995; 74:849–856.

Guthrie JF, Morton JF. Food sources of added sweeteners in the diets of Americans. *J Am Diet Assoc* 2000;100:43–51.

Hadjivassiliou M, Gibson A, Davies-Jones GA, Lobo AJ, Stephenson TJ, Milford-Ward A. Does cryptic gluten sensitivity play a part in neurological illness? *Lancet* 1996;347:369–371.

Hammond AC, Rumsey TS, Haaland GL. Prediction of empty body components in steers by urea dilution. *J Anim Sci* 1988;66:354–360.

Hanchette CL, Schwartz GC. Geographic patterns of prostate cancer mortality. Evidence for a protective effect of ultraviolet radiation. *Cancer* 1992;70: 2861–2869.

Harlan JR. The plants and animals that nourish man. *Sci Am* 1976;235:89–97.

Haskell WL. The influence of exercise on the concentrations of triglyceride and cholesterol in human plasma. *Exerc Sport Sci Rev* 1984;12:205–244.

Hawkes K, Hill K, O'Connell JF. Why hunters gather: optimal foraging and the Ache of eastern Paraguay. *Am Ethnologist* 1982;9:379–398.

Heal KG, Sheikh NA, Hollingdale MR, Morrow WJ, Taylor-Robinson AW. Potentiation by a novel alkaloid glycoside adjuvant of a protective cytotoxic T cell immune response specific for a preerythrocytic malaria vaccine candidate antigen. *Vaccine* 2001;19(30):4153–4161.

Hennekens CH, Buring JE. *Epidemiology in Medicine.* Boston: Little, Brown, 1987.

Hibbeln JR. Fish consumption and major depression. *Lancet* 1998;351:1213.

Hibbeln JR, Salem N. Dietary polyunsaturated fatty acids and depression: when cholesterol does not satisfy. *Am J Clin Nutr* 1995;62:1–9.

Hobbs CJ, Plymate SR, Rosen CJ, Adler RAI. Testosterone administration increases insulin-like growth factor-I levels in normal men. *J Clin Endocrinol Metab* 1993;77:776–779.

Hobbes T. *The Leviathan.* Amherst, NY: Prometheus Books, 1988.

Hochman LG, Scher RK, Meyerson MS. Brittle nails: response to daily biotin supplementation. *Cutis* 1993;51:303–305.

Hokanson JE, Austin MA. Plasma triglyceride level is a risk factor for cardiovascular disease independent of high-density lipoprotein cholesterol level: a meta-analysis of population-based prospective studies. *J Cardiovasc Risk* 1996;3: 213–219.

Holick MF. Vitamin D deficiency. *N Engl J Med* 2007;357:266–281.

Holly JMP. The physiological role of IGFBP-1. *Acta Endocrinol* 1991;124: 55–62.

Holmes MD, Stampfer MJ, Colditz GA, Rosner B, Hunter DJ, Willett WC. Dietary factors and the survival of women with breast carcinoma. *Cancer* 1999;86: 826–835.

Holt SH, Miller JB. Increased insulin responses to ingested foods are associated with lessened satiety. *Appetite* 1995;24:43–54.

Horner SM. Efficacy of intravenous magnesium in acute myocardial infarction in reducing arrhythmias and mortality. *Circulation* 1992;86:774–779.

Howell JM. Early farming in northwestern Europe. *Sci Am* 1987;257:118–126.

Hoyt G, Hickey MS, Cordain L. Dissociation of the glycaemic and insulinaemic responses to whole and skimmed milk. *Br J Nutr* 2005;93(2): 175–177.

Hu FB, Stampfer MJ, Manson JE, Rimm EB, Colditz GA, Speizer FE, Hennekens CH, Willett WC. Dietary protein and risk of ischemic heart disease in women. *Am J Clin Nutr* 1999;70:221–227.

Hu FB, Stampfer MJ, Rimm EB, Manson JE, Ascherio A, Colditz GA, Rosner BA, Spiegelman D, Speizer FE, Sacks FM, Hennekens CH, Willett WC. A prospective study of egg consumption and risk of cardiovascular disease in men and women. *JAMA* 1999;281:1387–1394.

Hung S, Umemura T, Yamashiro S, Slinger SJ. The effects of original and randomized rapeseed oils containing high or very low levels of erucic acid on cardiac lipids and myocardial lesions in rats. *Lipids* 1977;12(2): 215–221.

Hunter DJ, Willett WC. Diet, body size, and breast cancer. *Epidemiol Rev* 1993; 15:110–132.

Hwalla Baba N, Sawaya S, Torbay N, Habbal Z, Azar S, Hashim SA . High protein vs. high carbohydrate hypoenergetic diet for the treatment of obese hyperinsulinemic subjects. *Int J Obes* 1999;23:1202–1206.

Ip C, Scimeca JA, Thompson HJ. Conjugated linoleic acid. A powerful anticarcinogen from animal fat sources. *Cancer* 1994;74(suppl 3):1050–1054.

Is our fish fit to eat? *Consumer Reports* 1992(February);103–114.

Itami S, Kurata S, Takayasu S. Androgen induction of follicular epithelial cell growth is mediated via insulin-like growth factor-I from dermal papilla cells. *Biochem Biophys Res Commun* 1995;212:988–994.

Ivy JL. Role of exercise training in the prevention and treatment of insulin resistance and on insulin-dependent diabetes mellitus. *Sports Med* 1997; 24:321–336.

Jacobson MS. Cholesterol oxides in Indian ghee: possible cause of unexplained high risk of atherosclerosis in Indian immigrant populations. *Lancet* 1987; 2:656–658.

Jensen-Jarolim E, Gajdzik L, Haberl I, Kraft D, Scheiner O, Graf J. Hot spices influence permeability of human intestinal epithelial monolayers. *J Nutr* 1998;128:577–581.

Juul A, Scheike T, Nielsen CT, Krabbe S, Muller J, Skakkebaek NE. Serum insulin-like growth factor I (IGF-1) and IGF-binding protein 3 levels are increased in central precocious puberty: effects of two different treatment regimens with gonadotropin-relating hormone agonists, without or in combination with an antiandrogen (cyproterone acetate). *J Clin Endocrinol Metab* 1995; 80:3059–3067.

Kane J. *Savages.* New York: Random House, 1995.

Kelly RL. *The Foraging Spectrum. Diversity in Hunter-Gatherer Lifeways.* Washington, DC: Smithsonian Institution Press, 1995.

Key TJ, Fraser GE, Thorogood M, Appleby PN, Beral V, Reeves G, Burr ML, Chang-Claude J, Frentzel-Beyme R, Kuzma JW, Mann J, McPherson K. Mortality in vegetarians and nonvegetarians: detailed findings from a collaborative analysis of 5 prospective studies. *Am J Clin Nutr* 1999;70: 516S–524S.

Kinjo Y, Beral V, Akiba S, Key T, Mizuno S, Appleby P, Yamaguchi N, Watanabe S, Doll R. Possible protective effect of milk, meat and fish for cerebrovascular disease mortality in Japan. *J Epidemiol* 1999;9:268–274.

Klag MJ, Whelton PK. The decline in stroke mortality: an epidemiologic perspective. *Ann Epidemiol* 1993;3:571–575.

Klinger B, Anin S, Silbergeld A, Eshet R, Laron Z. Development of hyperandrogenism during treatment with insulin-like growth factor-I (IGF-I) in female patients with Laron syndrome. *Clin Endocrinol* 1998;48:81–87.

Knopp RH, Walden CE, Retzlaff BM, McCann BS, Dowdy AA, Albers JJ, Gey GO, Cooper MN. Long-term cholesterol lowering effects of 4 fat restricted diets in hypercholesterolemic and combined hyperlipidemic men: The Dietary Alternatives Study. *JAMA* 1997;278:1509–1515.

Kobayashi M, Sasaki S, Hamada GS, Tsugane S. Serum n-3 fatty acids, fish consumption and cancer mortality in six Japanese populations in Japan and Brazil. *Jpn J Cancer Res* 1999;90(9):914–921.

Kokkinos PF, Narayan P, Colleran JA, Pittaras A, Notargiacomo A, Reda D, Papademetriou V. Effects of regular exercise on blood pressure and left ventricular hypertrophy in African-American men with severe hypertension. *N Engl J Med* 1995;333:1462–1467.

Kopinski JS, Leibholz, Bryden WL. Biotin studies in pigs. Biotin availability in feedstuffs for pigs and chickens. *Br J Nutr* 1989;62:773–780.

Kris-Etherton PM, Taylor DS, Yu-Poth S, Huth P, Moriarty K, Fishell V, Hargrove RL, Zhao G, Etherton TD. Polyunsaturated fatty acids in the food chain in the United States. *Am J Clin Nutr* 2000;71(suppl 1): 179S–188S.

Krober T. *Ishi in Two Worlds. A Biography of the Last Wild Indian in North America.* Los Angeles: University of California Press, 1961.

Kubow S. Lipid oxidation products in food and atherogenesis. *Nutr Rev* 1993; 51:33–40.

Kurtz TW, Al-Bander HA, Morris RC. "Salt-sensitive" essential hypertension in men. Is the sodium ion alone important? *N Engl J Med* 1987;317: 1043–1048.

Kushi LH, Fee RM, Folsom AR, Mink PJ, Anderson KE, Sellers TA. Physical activity and mortality in postmenopausal women. *JAMA* 1997;277: 1287–1292.

Larsen CS. Reading the bones of La Florida. *Sci Am* 2000;282:80–85.

Larsen CS, Schoeninger MJ, van der Merwe NJ, Moore KM, Lee-Thorp JA. Carbon and nitrogen stable isotopic signatures of human dietary change in the Georgia Bight. *Am J Phys Anthropol* 1992;89:197–214.

Lee RB, Daly RH (eds.). *The Cambridge Encyclopedia of Hunters and Gatherers.* Cambridge, UK: Cambridge University Press, 1999.

Lee-Thorp J, van der Merwe NJ, Brain CK. Diet of *Australopithecus robustus* at Swartkrans from stable isotopic analysis. *J Hum Evol* 1994;27:361–372.

Legge AJ, Rowley-Conway PA. Gazelle killing in stone age Syria. *Sci Am* 1988; 257:88–95.

Legro RS. Polycystic ovary syndrome: current and future treatment paradigms. *Am J Obstet Gynecol* 1998;179(6 Pt 2):S101–S108.

Leitzmann MF, Stampfer MJ, Michaud DS, Augustsson K, Colditz GC, Willett WC, Giovannucci EL. Dietary intake of n-3 and n-6 fatty acids and the risk of prostate cancer. *Am J Clin Nutr* 2004;80(1):204–216.

Lemann J, Lennon EJ. Role of diet, gastrointestinal tract and bone in acid-base homeostasis. *Kidney Int* 1972;1:275–279.

Leonard WR, Robertson ML. Evolutionary perspectives on human nutrition: the influence of brain and body size on diet and metabolism. *Am J Hum Biol* 1994;6:77–88.

Lewin R. A revolution of ideas in agricultural origins. *Science* 1988;240: 984–986.

Liao F, Folsom AR, Brancati FL. Is low magnesium concentration a risk factor for coronary heart disease? The Atherosclerosis Risk in Communities (ARIC) Study. *Am Heart J* 1998;136:480–490.

Lieb CW. The effects on human beings of a twelve months' exclusive meat diet. *JAMA* 1929;93:20–22.

Lin X, Gingrich JR, Bao W, Li J, Haroon ZA, Demark-Wahnefried W. Effect of flaxseed supplementation on prostatic carcinoma in transgenic mice. *Urology* 2002;60(5):919–924.

Lindeberg S, Lundh B. Apparent absence of stroke and ischaemic heart disease in a traditional Melanesian island: a clinical study in Kitava. *J Intern Med* 1993;233(3):269–275.

Lindgren BF, Segovia B, Lassarre C, Binoux M, Gourmelen M. Growth retardation in constitutionally short children is related both to low serum levels of insulin-like growth factor-I and to its reduced bioavailability. *Growth Regul* 1996;6:158–164.

Lindseth G, Lindseth PD. The relationship of diet to airsickness. *Aviat Space Environ Med* 1995;66:537–541.

Lipkin M, Newmark HL. Vitamin D, calcium and prevention of breast cancer: a review. *J Am Coll Nutr* 1999;18(suppl 5):392S–397S.

Liu B, Lee HY, Weinzimer SA, Powell DR, Clifford JL, Kurie JM, Cohen P. Direct functional interaction between insulin-like growth factor–binding protein-3 and retionoid X receptor-alpha regulate transcriptional signaling and apoptosis. *J Biol Chem* 2000;275:33607–33613.

Liu S, Willett WC, Stampfer MJ, Hu FB, Franz M, Sampson L, Hennekens CH, Manson JE. A prospective study of dietary glycemic load, carbohydrate intake, and risk of coronary heart disease in U.S. women. *Am J Clin Nutr* 2000;71:1455–1461.

Long C, Alterman T. Meet the real free-range eggs. *Mother Earth News,* 2007, MotherEarthNews.com, www.motherearthnews.com/Real-Food/2007-10-01/Tests-Reveal-Healthier-Eggs.aspx.

Lopez-Bote CJ. Effect of free-range feeding on omega-3 fatty acids and alpha-tocopherol content and oxidative stability of eggs. *Anim Feed Sci Technol* 1998;72:33–40.

Lorenz K. Cereals and schizophrenia. *Adv Cereal Sci Technol* 1990;10:435–469.

Ludwig DS. Dietary glycemic index and obesity. *J Nutr* 2000;130:280S–283S.

Ludwig DS, Majzoub JA, Al-Zahrani A, Dallal GE, Blanco I, Roberts SB. High glycemic index foods, overeating, and obesity. *Pediatrics* 1999; 103:E26.

MacDonald ML, Rogers QR. Nutrition of the domestic cat, a mammalian carnivore. *Ann Rev Nur* 1984;4:521–562.

Mancilha-Carvalho JJ, Crews DE. Lipid profiles of Yanomamo Indians of Brazil. *Prev Med* 1990;19:66–75.

Mann NJ, Li D, Sinclair AJ, Dudman NP, Guo XW, Elsworth GR, Wilson AK, Kelly FD. The effect of diet on plasma homocysteine concentrations in healthy male subjects. *Eur J Clin Nutr* 1999;53:895–899.

Marean CW, Assefa Z. Zooarchaeological evidence for the faunal exploitation behavior of neanderthals and early modern humans. *Evol Anthropol* 1999; 8:22–37.

Marks BL, Rippe JM. The importance of fat free mass maintenance in weight loss programmes. *Sports Med* 1996;22:273–281.

Marmer WN, Maxwell RJ, Williams JE. Effects of dietary regimen and tissue site on bovine fatty acid profiles. *J Anim Sci* 1984;59:109–121.

Martin-Moreno JM, Willett WC, Gorgojo L, Banegas JR, Rodriguez-Artalejo F, Fernandez-Rodriguez JC, Maisonneuve P, Boyle P. Dietary fat, olive oil intake and breast cancer risk. *Int J Cancer* 1994;58:774–780.

Mason SLR, et al. Preliminary investigation of the plant macro-remains from Dolni Vestonice II, and its implications for the role of plant foods in Palaeolithic and Mesolithic Europe. *Antiquity* 1994;68:48–57.

Mathews-Roth MM, Krinsky NI. Effect of dietary fat level on UV-B induced skin tumors, and anti-tumor action of b-carotene. *Photochem Photobiol* 1984;40: 671–673.

Meat and Livestock Association of Australia (www.mla.com.au/).

Medeiros LC, Belden RP, Williams ES. Selenium content of bison, elk and mule deer. *J Food Sci* 1993;4:731–733.

Meneely GR, Battarbee HD. High sodium–low potassium environment and hypertension. *Am J Cardiol* 1976;38:768–785.

Mertz JR, Wallman J. Choroidal retinoic acid synthesis: a possible mediator between refractive error and compensatory eye growth. *Exp Eye Res* 2000;70: 519–527.

Metlapally R, Ki CS, Li YJ, Tran-Viet KN, Abbott D, Malecaze F, Calvas P, Mackey DA, Rosenberg T, Paget S, Guggenheim JA, Young TL. Genetic association of insulin-like growth factor-1 polymorphisms with high-grade myopia in an international family cohort. *Invest Ophthalmol Vis Sci* 2010. (Epub ahead of print.)

Meyer C, Mueller MF, Duncker GI, Meyer HJ. Experimental animal myopia models are applicable to human juvenile-onset myopia. *Surv Ophthalmol* 1999;44 (suppl 1):S93–S102.

Mezzano D, Munoz X, Martinez C, Cuevas A, Panes O, Aranda E, Guasch V, Strobel P, Munoz B, Rodriguez S, Pereira J, Leighton F. Vegetarians and cardiovascular risk factors: hemostasis, inflammatory markers and plasma homocysteine. *Thromb Haemost* 1999;81:913–917.

Mickleborough TD, Gotshall RW, Rhodes J, Tucker A, Cordain L. Elevating dietary salt exacerbates leukotrienes-dependent hypernea-induced airway obstruction in guinea pigs. *J Appl Physiol* in press.

Mikkelsen PB, Toubro S, Astrup A. Effect of fat-reduced diets on 24-hr energy expenditure: comparisons between animal protein, vegetable protein, and carbohydrate. *Am J Clin Nutr* 2000;72:1135–1141.

Miller GJ, Field RA, Riley ML. Lipids in wild ruminant animals and steers. *J Food Qual* 1986;9:331–343.

Miller MM. Low sodium chloride intake in the treatment of insomnia and tension states. *JAMA* 1945;129:262–266.

Miller WC, Koceja DM, Hamilton EJ. A meta-analysis of the past 25 years of weight loss research using diet, exercise or diet plus exercise intervention. *Int J Obes Relat Metab Disord* 1997;21:941–947.

Milton K. Primate diets and gut morphology: implications for hominid evolution. In: Harris M, Ross EB (eds.), *Food and Evolution*. Philadelphia: Temple University Press, 1987, pp. 93–108.

————. Diet and primate evolution. *Sci Am* 1993;269:86–93.

Moan J, Dahlback A, Setlow RB. Epidemiological support for an hypothesis for melanoma induction indicating a role for UVA radiation. *Photochem Photobiol* 1999;70:243–247.

Mokdad AH, Serdula MK, Dietz WH, Bowman BA, Marks JS, Koplan JP. The spread of the obesity epidemic in the United States, 1991–1998. *JAMA* 1999;282:1519–1522.

Moore WJ, Corbett ME. Distribution of dental caries in ancient British populations. I. Anglo-Saxon period. *Caries Res* 1975;9:163–175; IV. The 19th century. *Caries Res* 1976;10:401–414.

Morrow WJ, Yang YW, Sheikh NA. Immunobiology of the Tomatine adjuvant. *Vaccine* 2004 23;22(19):2380–2384.

Moseson M, Koenig KL, Shore RE, Pasternack BS. The influence of medical conditions and associated hormones on the risk of breast cancer. *Int J Epidemiol* 1993;22:1000–1009.

Movius HL. A wooden spear of third interglacial age from lower Saxony. *Southwest J Anthropol* 1950;6:139–142.

Munger RG, Cerhan JR, Chiu BC. Prospective study of dietary protein intake and risk of hip fracture in postmenopausal women. *Am J Clin Nutr* 1999;69: 147–152.

Must A, Spadano J, Coakley EH, Field AE, Colditz G, Dietz WH. The disease burden associated with overweight and obesity. *JAMA* 1999;282: 1523–1529.

Mutti DO, Zadnik K, Adams AJ. Myopia. The nature vs. nurture debate goes on. *Invest Ophthalmol Vis Sci* 1996;37:952–957.

Nam SY, Lee EJ, Kim KR, Cha BS, Song YD, Lim SK, Lee HC, Huh KB. Effect of obesity on total and free insulin-like growth factor (IGF)-1, and their relationship to IGF-binding protein (BP)-1, IGFBP-2, IGFBP-3, insulin, and growth hormone. *Int J Obes Relat Metab Disord* 1997;21:355–359.

National Center for Health Statistics. *The Third National Health and Nutrition Survey, 1988–94.* Washington, DC: U.S. Department of Health and Human Services, 2000.

Neel JV. Health and disease in unacculturated Amerindian populations. *Ciba Found Symp* 1977;49:155–177.

Nelson GJ, Schmidt PC, Kelley DS. Low-fat diets do not lower plasma cholesterol levels in healthy men compared to high-fat diets with similar fatty acid composition at constant caloric intake. *Lipids* 1995;30:969–976.

Nestler JE. Insulin regulation of human ovarian androgens. *Hum Reprod* 1997; 12(suppl 1):53–62.

Nieman DC. *Exercise Testing and Prescription. A Health Related Approach.* London: Mayfield Publishing, 1999.

Norrish AE, Skeaff CM, Arribas GL, Sharpe SJ, Jackson RT. Prostate cancer risk and consumption of fish oils: a dietary biomarker-based case-control study. *Br J Cancer* 1999;81(7):1238–1242.

Nuttall FQ, Gannon MC. Plasma glucose and insulin response to macronutrients in nondiabetic and NIDDM subjects. *Diabetes Care* 1991;14:824–838.

Obarzanek E, Velletri PA, Cutler JA . Dietary protein and blood pressure. *JAMA* 1996;275:1598–1603.

Obeid OA, Mannan N, Perry G, Iles RA, Boucher BJ. Homocysteine and folate in healthy east London Bangladeshis. *Lancet* 1998;352:1829–1830.

O'Bryne DJ, O'Keefe SF, Shireman RB. Low-fat monounsaturated-rich diets reduce susceptibility of low density lipoproteins to peroxidation ex vivo. *Lipids* 1998;33:149–157.

O'Dea K, Traianedes K, Ireland P, Niall M, Sadler J, Hopper J, De Luise M. The effects of diet differing in fat, carbohydrate, and fiber on carbohydrate and lipid metabolism in type 2 diabetes. *J Am Diet Assoc* 1989;89:1076–1086.

Odeleye OE, de Courten M, Pettitt DJ, Ravussin E. Fasting hyperinsulinemia is a predictor of increased body weight gain and obesity in Pima Indian children. *Diabetes* 1997;46(8):1341–1345.

Oh SY, Ryue J, Hsieh CH, Bell DE. Eggs enriched in omega-3 fatty acids and alterations in lipid concentrations in plasma lipoproteins and in blood pressure. *Am J Clin Nutr* 1991;54:689–695.

Ohara N, Naito Y, Nagata T, Tatematsu K, Fuma SY, Tachibana S, Okuyama H. Exploration for unknown substances in rapeseed oil that shorten survival time of stroke-prone spontaneously hypertensive rats. Effects of super critical gas extraction fractions. *Food Chem Toxicol* 2006; 44(7):952–963.

Ohara N, Naito Y, Nagata T, Tachibana S, Okimoto M, Okuyama H. Dietary intake of rapeseed oil as the sole fat nutrient in Wistar rats—lack of increase in plasma lipids and renal lesions. *J Toxicol Sci* 2008; 33(5):641–645.

Ohara N, Naito Y, Kasama K, Shindo T, Yoshida H, Nagata T, Okuyama H. Similar changes in clinical and pathological parameters in Wistar Kyoto rats after a 13-week dietary intake of canola oil or a fatty acid composition–based interesterified canola oil mimic. *Food Chem Toxicol* 2009; 47(1):157–162.

O'Keefe JH, Jr, Cordain L. Cardiovascular disease resulting from a diet and lifestyle at odds with our Paleolithic genome: how to become a 21st-century hunter-gatherer. *Mayo Clin Proc* 2004;79(1):101–108.

Oliver WJ, Cohen EL, Neel JV. Blood pressure, sodium intake and sodium related hormones in the Yanomamo Indians, a "no-salt" culture. *Circulation* 1975; 52:146–151.

Orengo IF, Black HS, Wolf JE. Influence of fish oil supplementation on the minimal erytherma dose in humans. *Arch Dermatol Res* 1992;284:219–221.

Oshida Y, Yamanouchi K, Hayamizu S, Nagasawa J, Ohsawa I, Sato Y. Effects of training and training cessation on insulin action. *Int J Sports Med* 1991;12:484–486.

Packard RR, Lichtman AH, Libby P. Innate and adaptive immunity in atherosclerosis. *Semin Immunopathol* 2009;31(1):5–22.

Paleodiet Page, The. What Hunter-Gatherers Ate (www.paleofood.com).

Pasquali R, Casimirri F, Vicennati V. Weight control and its beneficial effect on fertility in women with obesity and polycystic ovary syndrome. *Hum Reprod* 1997;12(suppl 1):82–87.

Penny D, Steel M, Waddell PJ, Hendy MD. Improved analyses of human mtDNA sequences support a recent African origin for *Homo sapiens*. *Mol Biol Evol* 1995;12:863–882.

Phinney SD, Bistrian BR, Evans WJ, Gervino E, Blackburn GL. The human metabolic response to chronic ketosis without caloric restriction: physical and biochemical adaptations. *Metabolism* 1983;32:757–768.

Piatti PM, Monti F, Fermo I, Baruffaldi L, Nasser R, Santambrogio G, Librenti MC, Galli-Kienle M, Pontiroli AE, Pozza G. Hypocaloric high-protein diet improves glucose oxidation and spares lean body mass: comparison to hypocaloric high-carbohydrate diet. *Metabolism* 1994;43: 1481–1487.

Pili R, Kruszewski MP, Hager BW, Lantz J, Carducci MA. Combination of phenylbutyrate and 13-cis retinoic acid inhibits prostate tumor growth and angiogenesis. *Cancer Res* 2001;61:1477–1485.

Pitts GC, Bullard TR. Some interspecific aspects of body composition in mammals. In *Body Composition in Animals and Man* (Publication 1598). Washington, DC: National Academy of Sciences, 1968, pp. 45–70.

Poikonen S, Puumalainen TJ, Kautiainen H, Burri P, Palosuo T, Reunala T, Turjanmaa K. Turnip rape and oilseed rape are new potential food allergens in children with atopic dermatitis. *Allergy* 2006;61(1):124–127.

Poikonen S, Rancé F, Puumalainen TJ, Le Manach G, Reunala T, Turjanmaa K. Sensitization and allergy to turnip rape: a comparison between the Finnish and French children with atopic dermatitis. *Acta Paediatr* 2009;98(2):310–315

Porrini M, Crovetti R, Riso P, Santangelo A, Testolin G. Effects of physical and chemical characteristics of food on specific and general satiety. *Physiol Behav* 1995;57:461–468.

Porrini M, Santangelo A, Crovetti R, Riso P, Testolin G, Blundell JE. Weight, protein, fat, and timing of preloads affect food intake. *Physiol Behav* 1997; 62:563–570.

Prentice AM. Manipulation of dietary fat and energy density and subsequent effects on substrate flux and food intake. *Am J Clin Nutr* 1998; 67(suppl 3):535S–541S.

Price TD, Petersen EB. A Mesolithic camp in Denmark. *Sci Am* 1987;256:113–121.

Prior IA, Davidson F, Salmond CE, Czochanska Z. Cholesterol, coconuts, and diet on Polynesian atolls: a natural experiment: the Pukapuka and Tokelau island studies. *Am J Clin Nutr* 1981;34(8):1552–1561.

Proctor CA, Proctor TB, Proctor B. Etiology and treatment of fluid retention (hydrops) in Meniere's syndrome. *Ear Nose Throat J* 1992;71:631–635.

Proud VK, Rizzo WB, Patterson JW, Meard GS, Wolf B. Fatty acid alterations and carboxylase deficiencies in the skin of biotin-deficient rats. *Am J Clin Nutr* 1990;51:853–858.

Puumalainen TJ, Poikonen S, Kotovuori A, Vaali K, Kalkkinen N, Reunala T, Turjanmaa K, Palosuo T. Napins, 2S albumins, are major allergens in oilseed rape and turnip rape. *J Allergy Clin Immunol.* 2006;117(2): 426–432.

Rajah R, Valentinis B, Cohen P. Insulin-like growth factor (IGF)-binding protein-3 induces apoptosis and mediates the effects of transforming growth factor-beta 1 on programmed cell death through a p53- and IGF-independent mechanism. *J Biol Chem* 1997;272:12181–12188.

Ramsden CE, Faurot KR, Carrera-Bastos P, Cordain L, De Lorgeril M, Sperling LS. Dietary fat quality and coronary heart disease prevention: a unified theory based on evolutionary, historical, global, and modern perspectives. *Curr Treat Options Cardiovasc Med* 2009;11(4):289–301.

Rayssiguier Y, Gueux E. Magnesium and lipids in cardiovascular disease. *J Am Coll Nutr* 1986;5:507–519.

Reaven GM. Syndrome X: 6 years later. *J Intern Med* 1994;236 (suppl 736):13–22.

————. Pathophysiology of insulin resistance in human disease. *Physiol Rev* 1995;75:473–486.

Reaven GM, Chen YD, Jeppesen J, Maheux P, Krauss RM. Insulin resistance and hyperinsulinemia in individuals with small, dense low density lipoprotein particles. *J Clin Invest* 1993;92:141–146.

Reinhold JG. High phytate content of rural Iranian bread: a possible cause of human zinc deficiency. *Am J Clin Nutr* 1971;24:1204–1206.

Remer T, Manz F. Potential renal acid load of foods and its influence on urine ph. *J Am Diet Assoc* 1995;95:791–797.

Reynolds RD. Bioavailability of vitamin B_6 from plant foods. *Am J Clin Nutr* 1988;48:863–867.

Richards MP, Hedges RM. Gough's cave and sun hole cave human stable isotopic values indicate a high animal protein diet in the British upper Paleolithic. *J Archaeol Sci* 2000;27:1–3.

Richards MP, Pettitt PB, Trinkaus E, Smith FH, Paunovic M, Karavanic I. Neanderthal diet at Vindija and Neanderthal predation: the evidence from stable isotopes. *Proc Natl Acad Sci USA* 2000;97:7663–7666.

Rifkin J. *Beyond Beef.* London: Thorsons, 1994.

Robinson J. *Why Grassfed Is Best.* Vashon, WA: Vashon Island Press, 2000.

Robinson SM, Jaccard C, Persaud C, Jackson AA, Jequier E, Schutz Y. Protein turnover and thermogenesis in response to high-protein and high carbohydrate feeding in men. *Am J Clin Nutr* 1990;52:72–80.

Roche HM. Dietary carbohydrates and triacylglycerol metabolism. *Proc Nutr Soc* 1999;58:201–206.

Rode A, Shephard RJ. Physiological consequences of acculturation: a 20 year study of fitness in an Inuit community. *Eur J Appl Physiol* 1994;69: 516–524.

Roe DA. *A Plague of Corn.* Ithaca, NY: Cornell University Press, 1973.

Roman SD, Clarke CL, Hall RE, Ian EA, Sutherland RL. Expression and regulation of retinoic acid receptors in human breast cancer cells. *Cancer Res* 1992;52:2236–2242.

Rostow WW. *The Great Population Spike and After.* New York: Oxford University Press, 1998.

Rudman D, DiFulco TJ, Galambos JT, Smith RB III, Salam AA, Warren WD. Maximal rates of excretion and synthesis of urea in normal and cirrhotic subjects. *J Clin Invest* 1973;52:2241–2249.

Ruff CB, Larsen CS, Hayes WC. Structural changes in the femur with the transition to agriculture on the Georgia coast. *Am J Phys Anthropol* 1984;64: 125–136.

Rustan AC, Nenseter MS, Drevon CA. Omega-3 and omega-6 fatty acids in the insulin resistance syndrome. Lipid and lipoprotein metabolism and atherosclerosis. *Ann NY Acad Sci* 1997;827:310–326.

Sabate J, Fraser GE, Burke K, Knutsen SF, Bennett H, Lindsted KD. Effects of walnuts on serum lipid levels and blood pressure in normal men. *N Engl J Med* 1993; 328:603–607.

Sanders TA. Growth and development of British vegan children. *Am J Clin Nutr* 1988;48:822–825.

Sargent JR, Tacon AG. Development of farmed fish: a nutritionally necessary alternative to meat. *Proc Nutr Soc* 1999;58:377–383.

Schaefer O. When the Eskimo comes to town. *Nutr Today* 1971;6:8–16.

Schaller GB, Lowther GR. The relevance of carnivore behavior to the study of early hominids. *Southwest J Anthropol* 1969;25:307–341.

Scholz D. Relations between myopia and school achievements, growth and social factors. *Offentl Gesundheitswes* 1970;32:530–535.

Scott MJ, Scott AM. Effects of anabolic-androgenic steroids on the pilosebaceous unit. *Cutis* 1992;50:113–116.

Sebastian A, Harris ST, Ottaway JH, Todd KM, Morris RC Jr. Improved mineral balance and skeletal metabolism in postmenopausal women treated with potassium bicarbonate. *N Engl J Med* 1994;330:1776–1781.

Seino Y, Seino S, Ikeda M, Matsukura S, Imura H. Beneficial effects of high protein diet in treatment of mild diabetes. *Hum Nutr Appl Nutr* 1983;37A: 226–230.

Semaw S, Renne P, Harris JW, Feibel CS, Bernor RL, Fesseha N, Mowbray K. 2.5-million-year-old stone tools from Gona, Ethiopia. *Nature* 1997;385: 333–336.

Shahid SK, Schneider SH. Effects of exercise on insulin resistance syndrome. *Coronary Artery Dis* 2000;11:103–109.

Shipman P. Scavenging or hunting in early hominids: theoretical framework and tests. *Am Anthropol* 1986;88:27–43.

Shiue HJ, Sather C, Layman DK. Reduced carbohydrate/protein ratio enhances metabolic changes associated with weight loss diet. *FASEB J* 2001;15(4 Pt 1): A301.

Sidossis LS, Mittendorfer B, Chinkes D, Walser E, Wolfe RR. Effect of hyperglycemia-hyperinsulinemia on whole body and regional fatty acid metabolism. *Am J Physiol* 1999;276(3 Pt 1):E427–E434.

Sidossis LS, Stuart CA, Shulman GI, Lopaschuk GD, Wolfe RR. Glucose plus insulin regulate fat oxidation by controlling the rate of fatty acid entry into the mitochondria. *J Clin Invest* 1996;98:2244–2250.

Sigal RJ, El-Hashimy M, Martin BC, Soeldner JS, Krolewski AS, Warram JH. Acute postchallenge hyperinsulinemia predicts weight gain: a prospective study. *Diabetes* 1997; 46:1025–1029.

Simoons FJ. The geographic hypothesis and lactose malabsorption. A weighing of the evidence. *Dig Dis* 1978;23:963–980.

Simoons FJ. Celiac disease as a geographic problem. In Walcher DN, Kretchmer N (eds.), *Food, Nutrition and Evolution*. New York: Masson Publishing, 1981, pp. 179–199.

Simopoulos AP. Omega 3 fatty acids in the prevention-management of cardiovascular disease. *Can J Physiol Pharmacol* 1997;75:234–239.

Singer P, Berger I, Luck K, Taube C, Naumann E, Godicke W. Long-term effect of mackerel diet on blood pressure, serum lipids and thromboxane formation in patients with mild essential hypertension. *Atherosclerosis* 1986;62:259–265.

Skov AR, Toubro S, Bulow J, Krabbe K, Parving HH, Astrup AI. Changes in renal function during weight loss induced by high vs. low-protein low-fat diets in overweight subjects. *Int J Obes Relat Metab Disord* 1999 23:1170–1177.

Skov AR, Toubro S, Ronn B, Holm L, Astrup A. Randomized trial on protein vs. carbohydrate in ad libitum fat reduced diet for the treatment of obesity. *Int J Obes* 1999;23:528–536.

Smith RN, Braue A, Varigos GA, Mann NJ. The effect of a low glycemic load diet on acne vulgaris and the fatty acid composition of skin surface triglycerides. *J Dermatol Sci* 2008;50(1):41–52.

Smith RN, Mann NJ, Braue A, Mäkeläinen H, Varigos GA. A low-glycemic-load diet improves symptoms in acne vulgaris patients: a randomized controlled trial. *Am J Clin Nutr* 2007;86(1):107–115.

Smith RN, Mann NJ, Braue A, Mäkeläinen H, Varigos GA. The effect of a high-protein, low glycemic–load diet versus a conventional, high glycemic–load diet on biochemical parameters associated with acne vulgaris: a randomized, investigator-masked, controlled trial. *J Am Acad Dermatol* 2007;57(2):247–256.

Solomon CG. The epidemiology of polycystic ovary syndrome. Prevalence and associated disease risks. *Endocrinol Metab Clin North Am* 1999;28:247–263.

Speechly DP, Buffenstein R. Appetite dysfunction in obese males: evidence for role of hyperinsulinaemia in passive overconsumption with a high fat diet. *Eur J Clin Nutr* 2000;54:225–233.

Speth JD. Early hominid hunting and scavenging: the role of meat as an energy source. *J Hum Evol* 1989;18:329–343.

Speth JD, Spielmann KA. Energy source, protein metabolism, and hunter-gatherer subsistence strategies. *J Anthropol Archaeol* 1983;2:1–31.

Sponheimer M, Lee-Thorp JA. Isotopic evidence for the diet of an early hominid *Australopithecus africanus*. *Science* 1999;283:368–370.

Stamler J, Caggiula A, Grandits GA, Kjelsberg M, Cutler JA. Relationship to blood pressure of combinations of dietary macronutrients. Findings of the multiple risk factor intervention trial. (MRFIT). *Circulation* 1996;94:2417–2423.

Stampfer MJ, Krauss RM, Ma J, Blanche PJ, Holl LG, Sacks FM, Hennekens CH. A prospective study of triglyceride level, low-density lipoprotein particle diameter, and risk of myocardial infarction. *JAMA* 1996; 276:882–888.

Stampfer MJ, Sacks FM, Salvini S, Willett WC, Hennekens CH. A prospective study of cholesterol, apolipoproteins, and the risk of myocardial infarction. *N Engl J Med* 1991;325:373–381.

Stanford CB, Wallis J, Mpongo E, Goodall J. Hunting decisions in wild chimpanzees. *Behaviour* 1994;131:1–18.

Steegers EP, Eskes TB, Jongsma HW, Hein PR. Dietary sodium restriction during pregnancy: a historical review. *Eur J Obstet Gynecol Reprod Biol* 1991;40:83–90.

Stefansson V. *The Fat of the Land.* New York: Macmillan Company, 1960.

Steiner PE. Necropsies on Okinawans. Anatomic and pathologic observations. *Arch Pathol* 1946;42:359–380.

Stewart P, Darvill T, Lonky E, Reihman J, Pagano J, Bush B. Assessment of prenatal exposure to PCBs from maternal consumption of Great Lakes fish: an analysis of PCB pattern and concentration. *Environ Res* 1999;80(2 Pt 2): S87–S96.

Stoll AL, Severus WE, Freeman MP, Reuter S, Zboyan HA, Diamond E, Cress KK, Marangell LB. Omega 3 fatty acids in bipolar disorder: a preliminary double-blind, placebo-controlled trial. *Arch Gen Psychiatry* 1999; 56:407–412.

Stoll BA. Western diet, early puberty, and breast cancer risk. *Breast Cancer Res Treat* 1998;49:187–193.

Stuart AJ. Mammalian extinctions in the late Pleistocene of northern Eurasia and North America. *Biol Rev* 1991;66:453–562.

Stubbs RJ, van Wyk MC, Johnstone AM, Harbron CG. Breakfasts high in protein, fat or carbohydrate: effect on within-day appetite and energy balance. *Eur J Clin Nutr* 1996;50:409–417.

Su HY, Hickford JG, Bickerstaffe R, Palmer BR. Insulin-like growth factor 1 and hair growth. *Dermatol Online J* 1999,(2):1.

Sweeten MK, Cross HR, Smith GC, Savell JW, Smith SB. Lean beef: impetus for lipid modifications. *J Am Diet Assoc* 1990;90:87–92.

Sweeten MK, Cross HR, Smith GC, Smith SB. Subcellular distribution and composition of lipids in muscle and adipose tissues. *J Food Sci* 1990;43–45.

Tanskanen A, Hibbeln JR, Tuomilehto J, Uutela A, Haukkala A, Viinamaki H, Lehtonen J, Vartiainen E. Fish consumption and depressive symptoms in the general population in Finland. *Psychiatr Serv* 2001;52:529–531.

Taylor CB, Peng SK, Werthessen NT, Tham P, Lee KT. Spontaneously occurring angiotoxic derivatives of cholesterol. *Am J Clin Nutr* 1979;32:40–57.

Teikari JM. Myopia and stature. *Acta Ophthalmol* 1987;65:673–676.

Teleki G. The omnivorous chimpanzee. *Sci Am* 1973;228:33–42.

Testart A. The significance of food storage among hunter-gatherers: residence patterns, population densities, and social inequalities. *Curr Anthropol* 1982; 23:523–537.

Teuteberg HJ. Periods and turning points in the history of European diet: a preliminary outline of problems and methods. In Fenton A, Kisban E (eds.), *Food in Change. Eating Habits from the Middle Ages to the Present Day.* Atlantic Highlands, NJ: Humanities Press, 1986, pp. 11–23.

Thiboutot DM. An overview of acne and its treatment. *Cutis* 1996;57:8–12.

Thieme H. Lower palaeolithic hunting spears from Germany. *Nature* 1997;385: 807–810.

Thierry van Dessel HJ, Lee PD, Faessen G, Fauser BC, Giudice LC. Elevated serum levels of free insulin-like growth factor I in polycystic ovary syndrome. *J Clin Endocrinol Metab* 1999;84:3030–3035.

Thresher JS, Podolin DA, Wei Y, Mazzeo RS, Pagliassotti MJ. Comparison of the effects of sucrose and fructose on insulin action and glucose tolerance. *Am J Physiol Regul Integr Comp Physiol* 2000;279:R1334–R1340.

Tobian L. High-potassium diets markedly protect against stroke deaths and kidney disease in hypertensive rats, an echo from prehistoric days. *J Hypertens* 1986;4(suppl):S67–S76.

————. Potassium and sodium in hypertension. *J Hypertens* 1988;6(suppl 4): S12–S24.

————. Salt and hypertension. *Hypertension* 1991;17(suppl I):I-52–I-58.

Tobian L, Hanlon S. High sodium chloride diets injure arteries and raise mortality without changing blood pressure. *Hypertension* 1990; 15:900–903.

Tong WM, Hofer H, Ellinger A, Peterlik M, Cross HS. Mechanism of antimitogenic action of vitamin D in human colon carcinoma cells: relevance for suppression of epidermal growth factor-stimulated cell growth. *Oncol Res* 1999;11:77–84.

Torrey JC, Montu E. The influence of an exclusive meat diet on the flora of the human colon. *J Infect Dis* 1931;49:141–176.

Travers SH, Labarta JI, Gargosky SE, Rosenfeld RG, Jeffers BW, Eckel RH. Insulin-like growth factor binding protein-I levels are strongly associated with insulin sensitivity and obesity in early pubertal children. *J Clin Endocrinol Metab* 1998;83:1935–1939.

Tripoli E, Giammanco M, Tabacchi G, Di Majo D, Giammanco S, La Guardia M. The phenolic compounds of olive oil: structure, biological activity and beneficial effects on human health. *Nutr Res Rev* 2005;18(1): 98–112.

Trowell H. Dietary fibre: a paradigm. In: Trowell H, Burkitt D, Heaton K, Doll R (eds.), *Dietary Fibre, Fibre-Depleted Foods and Disease.* New York: Academic Press, 1985, pp. 1–20.

Tucker KL, Hannan MT, Chen H, Cupples LA, Wilson PW, Kiel DP. Potassium, magnesium, and fruit and vegetable intakes are associated with greater bone mineral density in elderly men and women. *Am J Clin Nutr* 1999; 69:727–736.

Turner CG. Dental anthropological indicators of agriculture among the Jomon people of central Japan. *Am J Phys Anthropol* 1979;51:619–636.

Turner JC. Adaptive strategies of selective fatty acid deposition in the bone marrow of desert bighorn sheep. *Comp Biochem Physiol* 1979;62A: 599–604.

Tuyns A. Salt and gastrointestinal cancer. *Nutr Cancer* 1988;11:229–232.

Umemura T, Slinger SJ, Bhatnagar MK, Yamashiro S. Histopathology of the heart from rats fed rapeseed oils. *Res Vet Sci* 1978;25(3):318–322.

United States Census Bureau. Historical Estimates of World Population. www.census .gov/ftp/pub/ipc/www/worldhis.html.

Vieth R, Bischoff-Ferrari H, Boucher BJ, Dawson-Hughes B, Garland CF, Heaney RP, et al. The urgent need to recommend an intake of vitamin D that is effective. *Am J Clin Nutr* 2007;85:649–650.

Watkins BA: Dietary biotin effects on desaturation and elongation of ^{14}C-linoleic acid in the chicken. *Nutr Res* 1990;10:325–334.

Webster D, Webster G. Optimal hunting and Pleistocene extinction. *Hum Ecol* 1984;12:275–289.

Weller O. The earliest rock salt exploitation in Europe. A salt mountain in Spanish Neolithic. *Antiquity* 2002;76:317–318.

Willett WC. Is dietary fat a major determinant of body fat? *Am J Clin Nutr* 1998;67(suppl):556S–562S.

Willett WC, Ascherio A. Trans fatty acids: are the effects only marginal? *Am J Public Health* 1994;84:722–724.

Williams GC, Nesse RM. The dawn of Darwinian medicine. *Q Rev Biol* 1991;66: 1–22.

Wilson ME. Premature elevation in serum insulin-like growth factor-I advances first ovulation in rhesus monkeys. *J Endocrinol* 1998; 158:247–257.

Wing RR. Physical activity in the treatment of the adulthood overweight and obesity: current evidence and research issues. *Med Sci Sports Exerc* 1999;31: S547–S552.

Winterhalder B, Smith EA (eds). *Hunter-Gatherer Foraging Strategies. Ethnographic and Archaeological Analyses.* Chicago: University of Chicago Press, 1981, pp. 1–268.

Wolever TM, Bolognesi C. Prediction of glucose and insulin responses of normal subjects after consuming mixed meals varying in energy, protein, fat, carbohydrate and glycemic index. *J Nutr* 1996;126:2807–2812.

Wolfe BM. Potential role of raising dietary protein intake for reducing risk of atherosclerosis. *Can J Cardiol* 1995;11(suppl G):127G –131G.

Wolfe BM, Giovannetti PM. Short-term effects of substituting protein for carbohydrate in the diets of moderately hypercholesterolemic human subjects. *Metabolism* 1991;40:338–343.

Wolfe BMJ, Piche LA. Replacement of carbohydrate by protein in a conventional-fat diet reduces cholesterol and triglyceride concentrations in healthy normolipidemic subjects. *Clin Invest Med* 1999;22:140–148.

Wolmarans P, Benade AJ, Kotze TJ, Daubitzer AK, Marais MP, Laubscher R. Plasma lipoprotein response to substituting fish for red meat in the diet. *Am J Clin Nutr* 1991; 53:1171–1176.

Wong WW, Copeland KC, Hergenroeder AC, Hill RB, Stuff JE, Ellis KJ. Serum concentrations of insulin, insulin-like growth factor-I and insulin-like growth factor binding proteins are different between white and African American girls. *J Pediatr* 1999;135:296–300.

Wood B, Collard M. The human genus. *Science* 1999;284:65–71.

Yang Q, Mori I, Shan L, Nakamura M, Nakamura Y, Utsunomiya H, Yoshimura G, Suzuma T, Tamaki T, Umemura T, Sakurai T, Kakudo K. Biallelic inactivation of retinoic acid receptor B2 gene by epigenetic change in breast cancer. *Am J Pathol* 2001;158:299–303.

Yang YW, Sheikh NA, Morrow WJ. The ultrastructure of tomatine adjuvant. *Biomaterials* 2002;23(23):4677–4686.

Yang YW, Wu CA, Morrow WJ. The apoptotic and necrotic effects of tomatine adjuvant. *Vaccine* 2004;22(17–18):2316–2327.

Zambon D, Sabate J, Munoz S, Campero B, Casals E, Merlos M, Laguna JC, Ros E. Substituting walnuts for monounsaturated fat improves the serum lipid profile of hypercholesterolemic men and women. A randomized crossover trial. *Ann Intern Med* 2000;132:538–546.

Zhang J, Temme EH, Kesteloot H. Fish consumption is inversely associated with male lung cancer mortality in countries with high levels of cigarette smoking or animal fat consumption. *Int J Epidemiol* 2000; 29:615–621.

Zhu X, Wallman J. Opposite effects of glucagon and insulin on compensation for spectacle lenses in chicks. *Invest Ophthalmol Vis Sci* 2009;50(1): 24–36.

Zimmerman MR. The paleopathology of the cardiovascular system. *Texas Heart Inst J* 1993;20252–20257.

Zohary D. The progenitors of wheat and barley in relation to domestication and agricultural dispersal in the Old World. In Ucko PJ, Dimbleby GW (eds.), *The Domestication and Exploitation of Plants and Animals.* Chicago: Aldine Publishing, 1969, pp. 45–65.

Zouboulis CC, Xia L, Akamatsu H, Seltmann H, Fritsch M, Hornemann S, Ruhl R, Chen W, Nau H, Orfanos CE. The human sebocyte culture model provides new insights into development and management of seborrhoea and acne. *Dermatology* 1998;196:21–31.

Zvelebil M. Postglacial foraging in the forests of Europe. *Sci Am* 1986;254: 104–115.

Index